WHAT TO DO ABOUT
BITES AND STINGS
OF VENOMOUS ANIMALS

WHAT TO DO ABOUT BITES AND STINGS OF VENOMOUS ANIMALS

ROBERT E. ARNOLD, M.D.

COLLIER BOOKS
A Division of Macmillan Publishing Co., Inc.
NEW YORK

COLLIER MACMILLAN PUBLISHERS
LONDON

Macmillan Publishing Co., Inc.
866 Third Avenue, New York, N.Y. 10022
Collier-Macmillan Canada Ltd.

What to Do About Bites and Stings of Venomous Animals is also published in a hardcover edition by Macmillan Publishing Co., Inc.

Library of Congress Catalog Card Number: 72-77647

First Collier Books Edition 1973
SECOND PRINTING 1974
Printed in the United States of America

CONTENTS

CHAPTER ONE

OVERVIEW

IN THE UNITED STATES, the subject of poisonous animals is surrounded by a cloud of mystery. The average person is so repulsed by snakes, spiders, scorpions, stingrays, and the like that being bitten by one of them evokes fear— fear not only on the part of the victim and his friends but also on the part of the physician who is besieged by a horde of frightened individuals demanding that he "do something." Unfortunately, since the subject usually is not covered in standard medical texts, the physician must resort to using whatever he can find as a guideline—often a Merck manual or even an old outdoor magazine—and the results are usually chaotic.

Ever since the serpent beguiled Eve, venomous animals have been a hazard to man, and throughout recorded history, he has had an extraordinary interest in them and in the treatment of their bites. This is evidenced by the writings of the ancient Egyptians, Greeks, Romans, and Arabs. The oldest medical papers in existence—writings from Egypt, dating from 1600 B.C.—contain procedures to be used for bites. Twenty-five sections of Book V of the Seven Books of Paulus Aegineta, which Francis Adams translated and commented on in 1846, were about venomous animal bites and their treatment.

Despite the great interest, however, not much progress was made until 1664 when Francesco Redi demonstrated that toxins must be injected under the skin to be effective. Further progress was made by Silas Weir Mitchell, who, in a work published in 1860, first showed that snake venoms are complex proteins. This discovery was followed by the development of antivenom, which when used properly is the keystone in the successful treatment of severe bites. Nevertheless, today the problem of how to treat bites most effectively and efficiently still exists, because the information available to the physician resembles to an astonishing degree the medical literature of over 100 years ago, when anyone who had an opinion was free to express it.

In examining the current literature, I was amazed to find so much of it written by veterinarians, herpetologists, arenologists (spider men), and men in allied fields. It is no wonder that treatment varies so greatly, for the procedures these men advise often bear little, if any, similarity to each other. For example, the following have all been recommended: Use ice, don't use ice; use a tourniquet, never use a tourniquet; "cut and suck," don't "cut and suck"; kill the snake and bring it in, don't bring in the snake.

This book is written in the hope that it will remedy the situation. Its object is to assess the *medical* importance of venomous animals in the continental United States. It is not intended to be a book on venoms nor one on animals. In it, I will:

1. Emphasize the importance of victims' being treated by practicing medical doctors only. Treating poisonous animal bites is a medical problem, and it should not be handled by zoologists, herpetologists, or venom experts, any more than a heart attack or appendicitis should.

2. Stress the point that first aid is exactly that—first aid. Ninety-nine percent of the time this means get the victim to a doctor as quickly as possible; the less done to him, the better. To say the least, it is distressing for a physician

to be presented with a patient who has been unnecessarily mutilated, perhaps permanently, by a well-intentioned first-aider. Although I advocate certain first aid measures in the book, I do so only after a careful search of the literature.

3. Discuss only the fundamentals of proper treatment and the pertinent complications and how to avoid them.

I will not discuss:

1. The proper techniques of amputation, tracheostomy, debridement, skin flaps and grafts, blood transfusion, or using mechanical ventilators, assuming that physicians are familiar with these techniques.

2. The role of venomous animals as vectors, or reservoirs, of viral, rickettsial, and bacterial diseases.

3. The numerous venomous animals whose bites produce burning and itching, reactions which are common and do not usually result in the loss of a limb or life.

Table 1. Deaths from Bites and Stings of Venomous Animals in the United States for the Years 1960–1969

Rattlesnake		65
Water moccasin		1
Copperhead		2
Coral snakes		1
Snakes, not identified		36
Cobra (suicide)		1
Python (constriction)		1
Scorpion		6
Wasp		58
Bees		51
Yellowjacket		11
Undetermined insects		53
Portuguese man-of-war		1
Ticks (*dermacentor variabilis*)		8
Black widow spider		4
Spider, not identified		17
Ant		1
Animals, not coded		26
Hornet		2
Snake serum		1
Brown spider		6
	Snakes	107
	Others	237
	Total	344

The statistics quoted in Table 1 and throughout the text on the number of deaths resulting from the bites and stings of venomous animals and insects are for the years 1960–1969, and were obtained from the various health departments in the United States. The listing of animals and insects in the table is according to the International Classification of Diseases E927-E905. The data are presented exactly as they were received.

From the information, it is apparent that the majority of the deaths were due to bites and stings of animals that ordinarily are not lethal, such as bees and wasps. These deaths are presumed to be due to anaphylactic shock.

ANAPHYLACTIC SHOCK

Introducing a foreign protein into a human being is dangerous and should not be done lightly. Allergic reactions, ranging from hives to death, can and do follow, and they can occur within minutes. Each year in the United States about 600 deaths are ascribed to anaphylactic shock; an untold number of victims survive with prompt treatment.

CHAPTER TWO

INSECTS

Hymenoptera—Flying Insects

THE HYMENOPTERA includes bees, wasps, yellowjackets, hornets, and ants, and accounts for more deaths than any other group of animals. In a 1959 report on deaths from venomous animals for the years 1950–1954, Parrish noted that 40 percent of the deaths were from Hymenoptera as opposed to 33 percent from snakes and 18 percent from spiders (29). His data are approximately the same as I found for the years 1960–1969.

In general, Hymenoptera victims are older than victims of other bites, and death occurs much quicker. Whereas spider-bite victims usually live about 18 hours and snake-bite victims from 6–48 hours, Hymenoptera sting victims usually die within an hour.

Respiratory edema is the most common finding in autopsies on Hymenoptera victims. The edema, if severe enough, causes a drop in circulatory volume. A vascular engorgement or coronary occlusion has been described, and nervous system involvement with meningeal edema and damage to the white matter sometimes occurs.

PREVENTION

Obviously, the easiest way to avoid trouble is to avoid the insects. To do this, it is helpful to recognize the insects and their nests when possible.

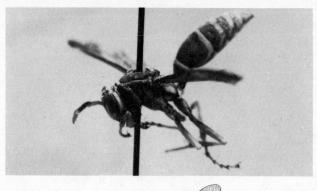

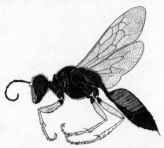

Wasps (Chlorion ichneumonea).
Note the very thin "waist." Color varies from orange to black, with many variations of stripes.

The paper wasp builds small paperlike honeycomb nests under eaves or in the rafters of garages, abandoned buildings, and the like. This wasp usually will not sting unless provoked, but it may become offensive.

The hornet lives in a large, round, paperlike nest hanging from trees or shrubs, or under eaves. Each nest may contain as many as 10,000 hornets which will attack in force at the slightest provocation.

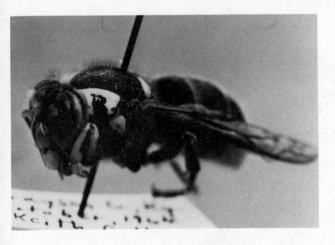

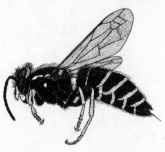

Hornets (Vespula maculata).
Fairly large—about one inch. Some body hair, but not as much as bees. The abdomen is predominantly black.

The yellowjacket is smaller than the wasp or hornet and has dark bands on its bright yellow body. It, too, builds a nest of paperlike material, but on the ground, especially along fence rows, or in logs. Since weeds and grass often hide the nests, they usually are found accidentally while cutting grass or walking through high weeds.

Bees, of course, generally are found in hives, although many stings are solitary, caused by stepping on bees that are gathering nectar.

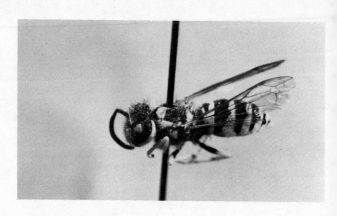

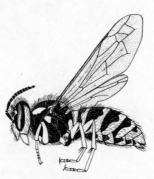

Yellowjackets (Vespula maculifrons).
Fairly small—½ to ¾ inch. The abdomen is much more yellow than in the hornet.

During the spring and summer months (there is no danger in cold weather), people who know they are allergic to insect venoms or who have other allergies would do well to follow these few simple rules when outdoors.

1. Keep away from scented preparations! Bees and wasps are attracted by the scents of deodorants, hair spray, and perfume.

2. Carry an aerosol insecticide spray. Keep it in the glove compartment of the car or, when outside, in a pocket or other handy place.

3. If you are extremely sensitive or have had previous anaphylactic reactions, you should carry a rapid-acting

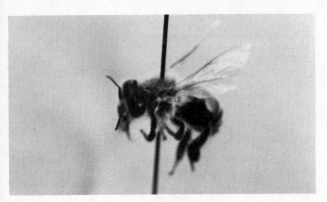

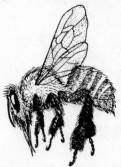

Bees (Apis mellifera).
Note the large legs. There is usually feathered hair on the body and legs, giving a fuzzy appearance.

antihistamine and a sprayer of epinephrine. A half dozen breaths from the sprayer and immediate ingestion of the antihistamine is very effective in thwarting anaphylactic reactions.

FIRST AID

If stung, do the following:

1. Remove the stinger if possible. The stinger looks like a small splinter and usually has a small venom sac attached. Generally it can be removed with a pointed knife, but be careful not to squeeze the venom into the skin when removing the stinger.
2. Apply ice to the sting. Cold tends to reduce chemical activity and also retards absorption of the venom.

A few hours of ice treatment should be sufficient. Avoid frostbite!

3. Get to a physician as quickly as possible if you are extremely allergy prone or have any of the following symptoms: shortness of breath, generalized edema (swelling), wheezing, abdominal pain, uterine cramps, fainting, or shock.

TREATMENT OF SEVERE REACTIONS

The immediate treatment of severe reactions to Hymenoptera stings is the same as that for other anaphylactic reactions.

1. Administer a 1:1000 solution of epinephrine very slowly intravenously.

2. Maintain an open airway. Sudden severe respiratory distress, indicated by a croup-like stridor, may arise secondary to laryngeal edema. To avert this, it will be necessary to do either an endotracheal intubation or, preferably, a tracheostomy.

3. Maintain the circulating blood volume. The edema may be severe enough to deplete the circulating blood volume with resulting hemoconcentration and shock. This will respond to intravenous fluids, preferably ringers lactate.

ANTIHISTAMINES AND CORTISONE

Antihistamines and cortisone are widely used in treating allergies and therefore deserve to be mentioned. For cases of mild urticaria (hives) and pruritis (itching), 50 mg. of diphenhydramine (Benadryl) or 4 mg. of chlorpheniramine maleate (Chlor-Trimeton) are useful. But in a severe attack, antihistamines are no substitute for epinephrine. Likewise, the late symptoms of anaphylactic shock may respond to cortisone, but cortisone is not fast acting enough to be useful in acute reactions. *Remember:* Epinephrine is the drug of choice for all anaphylactic reactions.

HYPOSENSITIZATION

Individuals who have a history of insect allergy should

be desensitized, especially in the summer months when working outside or planning a camping trip. The Insect Allergy Committee of the American Academy of Allergy recommends hyposensitization for systemic immediate-type reactions, and they have reported lessened reaction in 90 percent of the cases (17).

This very valuable procedure is simple. A commercial extract of bee, wasp, yellow jacket, and hornet bodies is prepared and injected in gradually increasing doses until the individual is able to tolerate as much venom as is in a normal sting without any reaction.

SUMMARY

Anaphylactic reactions from stings are the most common cause of deaths from venomous animals in the United States. Dramatic reversal of symptoms will usually be produced by administering epinephrine directly into the bloodstream, since death usually occurs very rapidly—the greatest number of victims die within 15–30 minutes, 88 percent die within 1 hour, and 96 percent within 5 hours (29). Victims with severe reactions should be taken to a doctor or hospital immediately. Removing the stinger, applying ice, and administering antihistamines are effective, but do not lose any time in getting the victim to a source of epinephrine. Do not wait for an ambulance or help to arrive.

HYMENOPTERA—ANTS

Ant stings may be painful. One death from ant sting has been reported. Some of the ants produce venom with properties similar to that of bees and wasps; others produce venom with more pronounced cholinergic properties. The fire ant of the southern United States causes a painful sting with vesicles and itching.

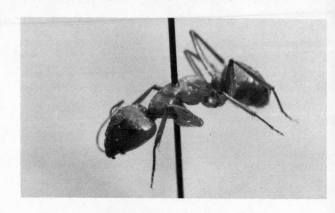

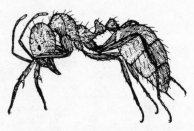

Fire Ants (Solenopsis geminata).
Note the thin body with two "bumps" in the center. There is some hair, and the legs are relatively long.

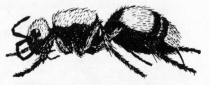

Velvet Ant (Mutilla sackeni).
Note the furry body, dark on the stomach and light on the back with dark stripes. Relatively short legs.

Other Insects

Assassin bugs, also called wheel bugs, are fairly common, and their salivary secretions are venomous. They inject venomous painful bites when handled, and although there have been no reports of deaths from them, there have been reports of anaphylactic reactions.

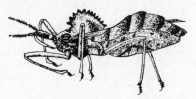

Assassin Bug (Wheel Bug) (Arilus cristatus).
Note the elongated body and well-developed wings. The "cog-wheel" crest on the thorax is distinctive.

Blister beetles (Spanish flies) deserve to be mentioned because of their supposed aphrodisiac powers. Cantharidin, a substance frequently taken in mistaken impression that it is an aphrodisiac, is present in the beetles' tissues, and crushing or handling the beetles will get the cantharidin on the skin, with blisters and superficial burns often resulting. Enough cantharidin can be absorbed through the skin to cause nephritis. It must be emphasized that cantharidin is *not* an aphrodisiac and when ingested it can cause severe kidney damage or death.

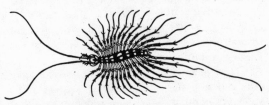

Eastern House Centipede (Scutigera cleoptrata).
Black or dark brown. Note the very long legs and antenna. Fairly rapid movement.

Centipedes are rather fast-moving wormlike creatures with fairly long legs. They are venomous and have heavy fangs to inject the venom. Mice and guinea pigs can be killed by centipedes, with death apparently due to respiratory failure and paralysis. Centipede bites in humans are characterized by immediate severe pain followed by red-

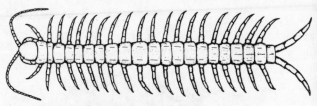

Western House Centipede (Scolopendra heros).
Black or dark brown. The body segments are hard and have one pair of legs each. The legs are shorter than those of the eastern house centipede, but longer than those of the millipede. Rapid movement.

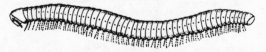

Millipede (Brachyiulus pussilus).
Brown color. Note the large, soft body and very short legs. Close inspection will reveal two pairs of legs per body segment. Very slow movement.

ness and swelling. Sometimes necrosis (tissue death) with ulcer formation may occur.

Millipedes are fairly common, slow-moving, large, rather soft worms with small legs. Their toxin is secreted by glands in the body. When the fluid touches the skin, it produces burning and itching. If the toxin gets into the eye, severe conjunctivitis results. In this case, wash the eye with large amounts of water.

Many caterpillars have hollow venom-containing hairs on their bodies. If these hairs contact the skin, they will cause severe burning pain, and redness, swelling, and necrosis may follow. Severe inflammation of the eyes may be caused by wind-blown hairs or touching the eyes with the fingers after touching a caterpillar.

Wash the eyes with copious amounts of water when inflamed. Scotch tape on the sting is very effective in removing broken spines. Severe generalized reactions will be benefited by intravenous calcium gluconate.

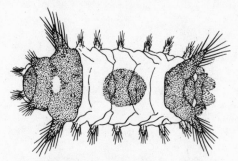

Saddleback Caterpillar (Sibine stimulae).
The "saddle" is distinctive. The body is soft. Slow movement.

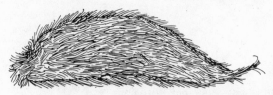

Puss Caterpillar (Megalopyge opercularis).
Soft body, covered with "fur."

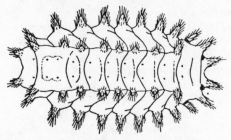

Slug Caterpillar (Euclea chloris).
About ¾ inch long. Color yellow-green.

TREATMENT

The treatment of these stings is very similar to that for Hymenoptera stings. Antihistamines, ice, and pain medication may be helpful. Epinephrine, of course, is indicated for anaphylactic-type reactions.

CHAPTER THREE

ARACHNIDS

Spiders

SPIDERS ARE THE MOST NUMEROUS, varied, and widespread of all the animals on the face of the earth. Thus far 100,-000 species have been identified. Spiders are found in the sky, in caves, on and under water, in deserts, forests, and mountains, in trees, grass, the ground, burrows, flowers, and practically any place on earth life is possible, with the exception of deep water. Spider populations are usually much larger than is apparent to the casual observer—spider counts have been reported to vary from 10,000 to 2,000,000 per acre.

Spiders are unobtrusive and usually the adjacent human world is largely unaware of their existence. They are small, eight-legged creatures with bodies that are divided into two parts, a cephalothorax (head and chest together) and a large baglike abdomen. The chelicera, or fangs, may be apparent or too small to be seen. They spend their entire lifetime (about a year) trapping and eating flies, mosquitoes, and other insects. Each spider is estimated to eat 2,000 insects in a lifetime. Spiders have almost no medical significance as carriers or vectors of disease. These last two facts make it apparent that spiders are probably the best friends man has in this world.

Practically all spiders produce venom (28), which is injected into trapped prey to kill and digest them. The spiders then suck their prey dry. Few spiders are venomous to man, for many reasons—the fangs are too weak to pierce skin or the gape is too narrow, the venom may not be particularly strong, or there is such a small amount of it that the effect is negligible. In spite of the fact that they do a great deal of good and very little harm, spiders are almost always feared and loathed. When noticed, they are usually killed for no reason at all.

Spider bites in the United States are common and the majority are not seen by a physician, nor do they require one. Although approximately 50 species of spiders have been implicated in human bites (16), severe reactions are usually limited to the *Latrodectus* and *Loxosceles* genera. For the years 1960–1969, 27 deaths from spider bites were reported. Of these, 4 were due to the black widow spider, 6 to "brown" spiders, and 17 to other spiders.

Latrodectus

Although species of the *Latrodectus* genus are found in every state in the United States and in Canada, they are less common in the north than in the south. Clinically significant species found in the United States are: *Latrodectus bishopi* (brown widow spider) in the southern states, *L. geometricus* (red widow spider) in Florida, *L. mactans hesperus* in the far western states, *L. mactans mactans* (black widow spider) in all the eastern states, and *L. mactans texanus* in the southwestern states (28).

Outdoor privies were once the classic examples of danger areas, but the disappearance of the outdoor privy has left the dumps, old lumber, and trash as the chief areas where man comes in contact with these spiders. The *Lactrodectus* are usually dangerous when accidentally squeezed or when their web is touched.

Deaths from *Lactrodectus* envenomation are rare at the present time. The deaths reported were in children and

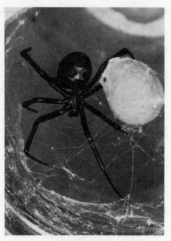

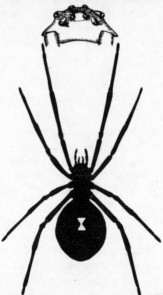

Black Widow Spiders (Latrodectus mactans mactans).
Fairly large—up to one inch long. Deep black with red "hourglass" on the abdomen. Eight eyes.

elderly people or from multiple bites. Victims with hypertension or heart trouble fared worse than others.

CLINICAL FINDINGS

In man, *Latrodectus* bites are painful. The initial pain is not severe, and two tiny red marks identify the site of entrance of the chelicera (fangs). Severe local pains follow and become very severe in about 30 minutes. The pain gradually spreads over the entire body and settles in the abdomen and legs. Sweating, salivation, nausea, vomiting, and a rash have been reported. The progression of symptoms is fairly rapid and coma may result in 30 minutes. The symptoms begin to regress in several hours, and usually are gone in a few days.

Latrodectus venom causes no tissue necrosis. The bite sites are prone to infection, probably due to the bacteria carried by the spider. Cellulitis, lymphangitis, and tetanus may follow. The venom has a primary neurotoxic effect, with the action apparently at the spinal cord or neuromuscular junction. An elevated cerebrospinal fluid pressure with hypertension is noted. The pain in the abdomen or chest is severe with no evidence of visceral involvement, that is, peristalsis is present. Many victims have not seen the spider and the diagnosis is made on the clinical picture.

TREATMENT

Morphine or meperidine (Demerol) is safe to use to relieve pain. Alcohol is harmful and should not be used. A solution of calcium gluconate is very effective in relieving pain, muscle spasm, and hypertension. Muscle relaxants are very effective. The use of methocarbamol (Robaxin) has been recommended as follows (35): One 10 cc. vial is given slowly intravenously over a 5 or 10 minute period, followed by 250 cc. of d5W (5 percent dextrose in water) with 10 cc. of methocarbamol added to run over a 4-hour period. For the next 24 hours, 80 mg of methocarbamol is given by mouth every 6 hours.

A specific antivenin effective against all *Latrodectus* venom is manufactured by Merck, Sharpe & Dohme Drug Company. The trade name is Lyovac, and it is a horse serum preparation. One unit of antivenin is reconstituted and added to 500 cc. of d5W and is then given intravenously in the next several hours. The usual skin test to prevent a horse serum reaction is of course necessary. Marked improvement is usually noted within 3 or 4 hours of administration.

Tetanus prophylaxis is necessary, as are antibiotics to prevent infections at the site of the bite.

Loxosceles

The *Loxosceles* genus of spiders is fairly widespread in the United States. These spiders are usually thought to be limited to the western states, but they have been identified in the eastern states, and there have been reports of bites from them in the east. Species commonly found in the United States are: *Loxosceles reclusa* in the southern and central states, *L. arizonica* in the southwestern states, *L. devia* in south Texas, and *L. unicolor* in the western states.

The most familiar species is *L. reclusa*, the brown recluse spider. The other species of this genus are not technically the brown recluse, but I will use this term to include all *Loxosceles* species. The brown recluses are small- to medium-sized spiders with a violin-shaped mark on their backs. They live in abandoned houses, cellars, and barns and in grass and cliffs. Infrequently used vacation cabins are often infested.

CLINICAL FINDINGS

Bites of the brown recluse spider do not constitute an emergency. There is no pain or so little pain that most of the time, the victim is not aware that he is bitten. A few

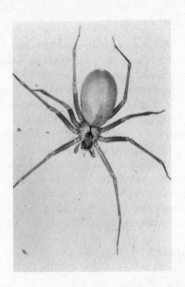

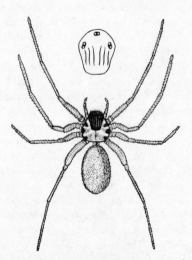

Brown Recluse Spiders (Loxosceles reclusa).
Light brown color. Small and delicate—usually less than ½ inch long. Note the narrow waist and the dark brown "violin" on the back.

hours later a painful, red area with a mottled cyanotic center appears. A morbilliform macular rash sometimes occurs. Necrosis does not occur in all bites, but usually after 2 or 3 days inpending necrosis is evident in an area of discoloration that does not blanch with finger pressure. The center becomes indurated, and there is marked surrounding erythema. The central ischemia becomes stellate, and the area turns dark and becomes mummified in a week or two. The margins separate and the eschar falls off leaving an open ulcer (25). The edges of the ulcer are undermined because the toxin has more effect on the superficial fascia than on the skin. Secondary infection and regional lymphadenopathy usually become evident at this stage. This is the point at which most bites are first seen by a physician. Many times the patient is unaware of any cause for this ulcer, and there is little on examination to distinguish this bite from any other.

Many other insect and arthopod bites cause local necrosis, most notably the venomous tick, the pajaroello. It is entirely possible that many bites ascribed to brown recluse spiders may actually be from some other insect. Clinically, the outstanding feature of brown recluse bites is that the ulcer does not heal, but persists for weeks or months. Physical examination reveals a hard indurated area of skin and superficial fascia with undermined edges.

In many cases there is a systemic reaction in addition to the ulcer. Systemic reactions are serious and may lead to death. They occur chiefly in children (25) and are marked by fever, chills, joint pain, splenomegaly, vomiting, and a generalized rash. Intravascular hemolysis and thrombocytopenia also occur—the hemoglobin and hematocrit are down and the bilirubin is elevated with hemoglobiuria (dark urine). Systemic reactions may occur at any time as long as the ulcer is present.

TREATMENT

There is no specific antivenin for brown recluse bites.

Since the toxin remains in the fascia for a long time, it is necessary to excise the bite before healing will occur. All the indurated skin and fascia must be excised (48). When this infecting source is removed, the patient's condition improves rapidly and the ulcer begins to heal. Should this necrotic ulcer not be excised, it may continue to grow until it is several inches in diameter.

Cortisone will arrest the systemic reaction, but it will not effect the necrotic ulcer (25). Blood transfusions as well as antibiotics may be necessary to control secondary infections. Tetanus prophylaxis is, of course, mandatory. Since renal shutdown may follow intravascular hemolysis, dialysis may be necessary.

South American Species

South America is the home of a brown spider, *Loxosceles laeta*, which produces a very toxic venom. The venom produces marked tissue destruction with necrosis, and the ulcers will rot away to the bone. Treatment includes debridement and cortisone, if a systemic reaction is encountered. A specific antivenom is commercially available in South America and is very effective.

Other Spiders

Many people who are bitten by spiders go to their local physicians with many and varied complaints. A single case of mild symptoms from the bite of the common garden spider (*Cheiracanthium inclusam*) has been reported. The local painful reaction disappeared in 12 hours. The tarantulas are fearsome looking but not very dangerous.

Scorpions

Scorpions are the most feared venomous animals in certain endemic areas. The Book of Revelations predicts a scourge of locusts with the power of scorpions in the last days. The scourge is to last five months, "and to them it was given that they should not kill them, but their torment was as the torment of a scorpion, when he striketh a man. And in those days shall men seek death and not find it" (15).

There are six families and 600 species of scorpions. They are usually larger and more poisonous in hot dry climates, such as in North Africa, the Middle East, and Mexico, and they are well adapted to life on the desert. Nearly all the very poisonous species belong to the family Buthidae, which fortunately is not found in the United States (18).

Scorpions have eight legs and pincers and superficially resemble a small crab with a tail arched over its back. All scorpions are venomous. The tip of the tail contains the stinger or telson which injects the venom. Stings occur more frequently during periods of rain or high humidity, and most of them are on the hands and feet.

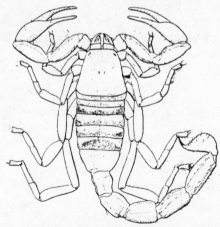

Hairy Scorpion (Hadrurus arizonensis).
Olive gray color. Fairly large, with many hairs on the body and stinger—more than the drawing shows. The sting is painful, but the venom is relatively weak, and no deaths have been reported from it.

The large hairy scorpion, *Hadrurus arizonensis*, has a very painful sting with swelling but very little systemic reaction. No fatalities from this scorpion have been recorded. I personally feel that this is the most repulsive looking and fearsome animal I have seen. Many other scorpions have stripes on their backs or are completely black. These are usually not very venomous. The sting of sculptured scorpion, on the other hand, can be fatal. This scorpion has a yellow back with no stripes, a small bump just beneath the stinger. Check for this with a magnifying glass after the scorpion is dead.

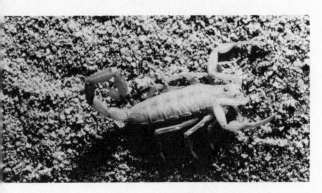

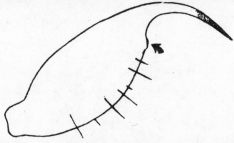

Sculptured Scorpions (Centruroides sculpturatus).
Identification is important, as the sting may be fatal. The distinctive features are: (1) yellow color, with no stripes or other colors; (2) relatively few hairs; (3) subaculear tooth beneath the stinger—may be difficult to see without magnification.

For the years 1960–1969, six deaths from scorpion stings were reported in the United States—four in Arizona, one in Texas, and one in Florida. Several insects are similar to scorpions and in haste may be mistaken for them. The pictorial keys are helpful in distinguishing these.

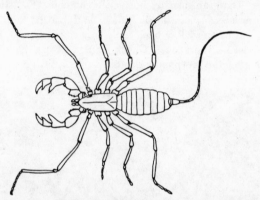

Whip Scorpion (Trithyreus pentapeltis).
Yellow color. Note the relatively small claws and long legs. The tail has no stinger, but is whipped about, spraying an irritating venom.

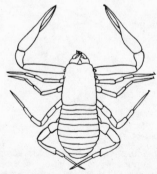

Pseudoscorpion (Chelifer cancroides).
May be confused with scorpions at first glance, but has no tail and no stinger.

PREVENTION OF BITES

How to prevent scorpion bites can best be summarized in one sentence—Watch your hands and feet! In endemic areas, the following precautions should be taken.

1. Wear heavy work gloves when cleaning up debris, and pick up boards and look on the underside of them instead of blindly sticking your fingers under them. A favorite habitat of scorpions is on the underside of scrap lumber and debris.

2. Use a good pesticide in yards and lumber piles.

3. If you feel something crawling over your body in the dark, do not swat it; brush it off. Swatting will guarantee envenomation, but a quick brush will remove the scorpion before it can sting (27).

4. Check clothing and shoes before putting them on.

FIRST AID

Get to a doctor or hospital! Hypothermia (cooling) has been reported to be beneficial, but must be started at once. Hypothermia retards absorption of venom and is beneficial for about 15–30 minutes. Place hand or foot in a large vessel of ice water while going to the hospital. If possible bring the scorpion to the doctor or hospital for it is very helpful if the species is identified.

CLINICAL FINDINGS

Scorpions in the United States may be placed in two clinical groups (27). The first group, which includes all but two species, produces a severe local reaction. Pain and swelling is marked with ecchymosis. Tissue slough is usually not a problem. Prickly sensations around the mouth and a thick tongue have been reported.

The second group, which includes *Centuroides sculpturatus Ewing* and *Centuroides gerstschi Stahnke*, produces a severe systemic reaction and very little or no visible local reaction. Local pain and hyperesthesia may be present. The systemic effects are respiratory difficulties, thick tongue, or opisthotonic spasms, drooling, gastric distention, diplopia, blindness, mystagmus, involuntary micturition, and defecation, penile erection, hypertension, and heart failure (44). Death is rare, occurring chiefly in children or adults with hypertension.

TREATMENT

Paraldehyde and morphine and morphine derivatives, including meperidine (Demerol), are contraindicated because these drugs have a synergistic effect with scorpion venom (44). Effective pain relief can be obtained with specific nerve blocks. Axillary block or specific nerve block in the upper extremity with lidocaine (Xylocaine) is safe and effective. Nerve blocks to the lower extremity are more difficult but effective if done carefully.

A specific antivenin for *Centruroides sculpturatus* is available. It is a goat serum manufactured by the Poisonous Animals Research Laboratory in Tempe, Arizona. The usual therapeutic dose is 3 cc. in 500 cc. d5W given slowly intravenously. Antivenin is available at most hospitals and doctor's offices in Arizona. In case of emergencies in other states, contact the Poisonous Animals Research Laboratory Tempe, Arizona, Monday thru Friday, 8:00 A.M.–4:30 P.M., (telephone 602-965-3536). At other times the security department could locate the director if necessary (telephone 602-965-3456).

Tetanus prophylaxis and broad spectrum antibiotics are indicated.

Mexican Species

Scorpions kill more people in Mexico than all other animals combined. In the years 1940–1949, scorpion sting caused 1588–1944 deaths a year. These occurred mostly in the dry western states of Colima, Mayarit, Guerrero and Morelos. A specific antivenin is commercially available in Mexico and in all hospitals for the scorpions found in these states. The antivenin manufactured by the Poisonous Animals Research Laboratory is not recommended, although it may be beneficial.

Ticks

Ticks are found in damp areas, grass, and weeds. They are attracted to the edges of paths, probably by the scent of animal odors. They lurk here ready to attach themselves

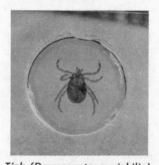

Tick (Dermacentor variabilis).
Note the small, rounded body, with eight legs. The size of the body varies greatly according to the amount of blood in the stomach—may be ¼ to ½ inch long. The legs appear smaller when the tick is engorged.

to any passing host. The tick season starts in March and ends in August, with the peak in May, June, and July.

Tick paralysis in man is fairly rare and inconstant. Eight deaths from tick paralysis have been reported in the years 1960–1969. However, sheep are commonly affected and cattle and dogs occasionally (44). The disease is usually associated with *Dermacentor variabilis* and *Dermacentor andersoni*, but other ticks have also been implicated. The disease is transmitted by means of a toxin secreted by the pregnant female. After she lays her eggs, the female loses her toxicity.

Children, generally under 10 years of age, are usually affected, but there have been a few cases in elderly people. The onset of symptoms begins 9 to 16 days after attachment, corresponding to the time of engorgement. The symptoms are much worse when the tick is attached to the neck and spinal column, and they are very severe in children under 2 years of age.

When camping in areas where ticks abound, children, dogs, and even adults should be deticked twice a day. This will effectively prevent tick paralysis.

CLINICAL FINDINGS

The disease is a progressive, ascending, flaccid, motor paralysis. Microscopically there is extensive destruction of myelin sheaths. Initial manifestations usually include irritability, lack of appetite, and pain or numbness in the legs. Within the next 24 hours lower back muscles are affected so the victim can no longer sit up, and then the upper extremities are affected. The patient becomes apathetic but remains conscious. Speech becomes impaired, then swallowing, and finally respiratory paralysis will occur. This clinical picture will be reversed at any stage by removing the tick.

In 1954, Rose reviewed 322 recorded cases of tick paralysis and found a mortality rate of 11.7% (33). This seems extremely high considering the simplicity of treatment. He found that cases with a fatal outcome usually occurred in three groups: (a) those not seen by a doctor (b) those seen by a doctor but in the terminal stages, and (c) those under medical care, but an incorrect diagnosis was made.

DIAGNOSIS

The diagnosis of tick paralysis can only be made if the physician keeps the possibility in mind in any case of ascending paralysis, especially from February to August. This diagnosis should be considered too in areas where ticks ordinarily do not occur since the latent period between attachment of the tick and the onset of symptoms is long enough to permit the patient to travel out of an edemic area before becoming ill.

Clinically it is very important to distinguish this disease from polio. The disease occurs in the hot summer months, and is very similar to polio. The following will help in distinguishing tick paralysis from polio (10).

1. Absence of fever
2. Ascending paralysis which is relatively painless, symmetrical, and flaccid
3. Normal spinal fluid
4. Absence of particular pain or spasm
5. Deep reflexes lost early, before paralysis
6. Extreme apathy
7. Finding a tick

A mild type of paralysis may occur and is characterized by slight weakness of the extremities and a cerebellar type of ataxia.

TREATMENT

1. Find the tick. Look carefully in hairy areas, such as scalp, eyebrows, axillae and perineum. Remember that more than one tick may be present. An engorged tick (10 mm. x 13 mm.) resembles a wart or fibroma and may be mistaken for one.

2. Remove of the tick. The tick must be removed in one piece. One death has been attributed to leaving the mouth parts behind. Put a drop of ether, gasoline or benzene on the tick, touch it with a lit cigarette, or bury it in petrolatum. Wait at least 10 minutes and attempt to pull the tick off. If this fails, excise a small piece of skin with the tick attached (7).

3. Supportive treatment may require intravenous fluids, tracheotomy to control secretions, and a mechanical ventilator. There is no antivenin available, but the disease is rapidly reversible.

CHAPTER FOUR

MARINE ANIMALS

THE OCEANS AND SEAS of the world account for approximately 75 percent of the earth's surface. Eighty-five percent of all life on earth exists in the sea, and this life is in a constant state of flux or change. As is true of all life, marine life is organized into a food chain. At the bottom of the chain are the diatoms, the grass of the ocean, which are fed on by the larger plankton. These, in turn are fed on by slightly larger animals, and so on up the chain. At the end of the feeding line are the many fishes, eels, and so forth with which we are familiar. In this food chain, the size of the animal increases from one link to the next. Obviously, the larger animals are safer since there are fewer animals capable of eating them, but they, in turn, require more food to stay alive. Many of these animals have developed toxins for feeding or defensive purposes.

Although there are approximately 1000 species of venomous or poisonous marine animals, and the venoms they produce are as varied as those produced by land-dwelling animals, the discussion that follows will be limited to the venomous animals commonly found in the North American coastal waters.

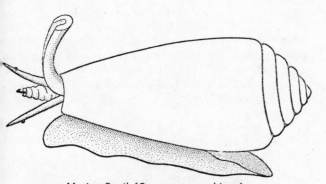

Marine Snail (Conus geographicus).
A large venom sac is attached to a barbed stinger carried in the mouth.

Snails, Sea Urchins, and Corals

The marine snails of the genus *Conus* are venomous. The venom is injected with a harpoon-like tooth. Shell collectors seem to suffer the most from these snails. The milder cases of envenomation resemble bee or wasp stings. More severe symptoms are fairly severe pain, followed by numbness, paresthesia (tingling sensation), paresis (partial paralysis) that may involve the entire skeletal musculature, difficulty in swallowing, a sense of constriction of the chest, visual disturbance, and collapse. The deaths recorded have been associated with *C. geographicus* in the South Pacific and Indian Oceans. There have been no fatalities in North American waters. There is no known antivenin and treatment is entirely symptomatic.

The spines of sea urchins cause painful injuries, dizziness, and muscular palsies, lasting for several hours. Hydroids, sea anemones, and stinging corals cause stinging with hemorrhagic lesions that may lead to necrosis. Severe stings may produce abdominal cramps, chills, diarrhea, and an elevated white blood cell count. There is no specific treatment for these usually minor injuries.

Scorpion Fish

The scorpion fish are the most dangerous poisonous fishes in North American waters. The venom glands are associated with the spines, especially on the dorsal fins. These are shallow water fish, generally found around reefs and coral, where they stay in crevices. Each year about

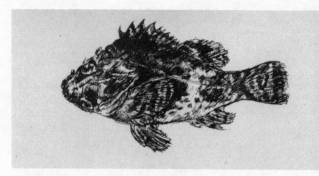

Scorpion Fish (Scorpaena guttata).

300 people are stung by scorpion fish (38), but no deaths have been reported. Scuba divers are usually injured by accidentally stepping on or touching them, and fishermen are injured when removing them from nets and traps.

Envenomation causes local, usually intense pain which spreads and is accompanied by swelling, blistering, and local necrosis of tissue. Victims commonly become hyperactive, and they may roll around on the ground in agony. Systemic symptoms are marked sweating, shortness of breath, shock, and cyanosis. Victims may complain of weakness, muscular aches, and shortness of breath for weeks.

TREATMENT

Immersing the injured part in hot water affords relief, since heat deactivates the venom. A solution of emetine hydrochloride (65 mg. per cc.) infiltrated around the wound may be beneficial. An antivenom is available. The antivenom is made from the venom of *Synanceja verrucosa*, a very dangerous fish found in the South Pacific. A dose of 2 cc. is given intravenously and may be repeated as needed.

Stingrays

Stingrays are common in coastal waters. They may reach a size of 8–10 feet in length and may weigh as much as 100 pounds. The venom is secreted on the bony spines on the dorsum of the tail, which may be as long as 16 inches. Stingrays bury themselves in sand or mud. When the vic-

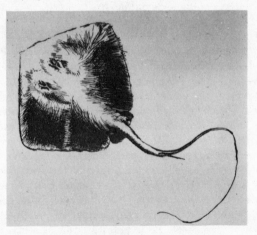

Stingray (Dasyatis longus).

tim steps on the stingray, it lashes out its tail, stinging the victim. Large stingrays may drive the stinger into the chest or abdomen.

About 750 people are stung by stingrays each year, and although there have been deaths reported, they are rare.

Initially there is usually a zone of blanching around the wound, followed by redness and swelling. There is severe pain accompanied by nausea, sweating, and fainting. Severe wounds cause convulsions, irregular breathing, and cardiac arrythmias.

TREATMENT

Treatment consists of debriding and cleaning the wound. All pieces of spine and sheath should be removed, and the envenomated part should be immersed in hot water for 30–90 minutes to deactivate the toxin. There is no antivenom available.

Jellyfish

During the ten year period 1960–1969, only one death from a Portugese man-of-war sting was reported. Parrish noted that two deaths were reported during the years 1950–1954. The Portugese man-of-war is a siphonophore and lives at the actual surface of the sea. It resembles a glob of clear bluish jelly floating on the surface of the sea. Long threadlike tentacles studded with toxin-containing nematocysts hang down in the water.

The jellyfish, of course, cannot attack man. The unfortunate victim usually swims into the tentacles. Contact with the tentacles causes severe, intense pain. Lines are evident where the tentacles have touched. Systemic reactions include muscular cramps, shortness of breath, nausea, weakness, and shock. Local necrosis of the skin may occur.

TREATMENT

Treatment consists of first applying alcohol or ammonia to deactivate the toxin-containing nematocysts and then applying flour or sand and scraping it off. The dry material adheres to the tentacles and makes it easier to remove them. Analgesic creams are beneficial, and antihistamines are indicated.

Systemic reactions can be treated effectively with epinephrine and calcium gluconate. The epinephrine may be given intramuscularly or subcutaneously unless the victim is in shock, in which case small increments must be given intravenously (39). A 10 cc. dose of calcium gluconate administered intravenously is usually sufficient. Morphine or meperidine (Demerol) are both safe to give for pain relief.

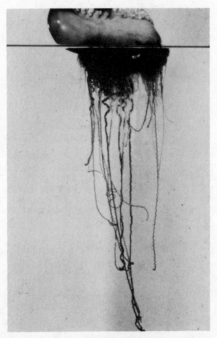

Portugese Man-of-War (Physalia arethusa).
The float is about eight inches long. The tentacles, which are difficult to see when swimming or scuba diving, may be as long as sixty feet.
PHOTOGRAPH COURTESY OF U.S. PUBLIC HEALTH SERVICE.

Sea Snakes

There are about 50 species of sea snakes in the world, and fortunately they are found predominantly in the South Pacific. Since eels and lampreys have been mistaken for sea snakes in the past, a word of reassurance is in order here. The Atlantic Ocean is free of sea snakes!

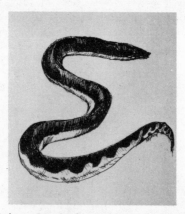

Pelagic Sea Snake (Pelamis platurus).
Black or brown with a yellow belly and a lateral stripe. The tail is mottled. Nostrils are often at the top of the head. The paddle-shaped tail markedly increases their ability to swim, but they are awkward on land. Easily distinguished from eels by lack of fins or gill openings and presence of scales.
DRAWING COURTESY OF U.S. PUBLIC HEALTH SERVICE.

Land snakes, notably the eastern diamondback rattlesnake, can swim, and frequently do to the offshore islands along the southeastern coastal United States. The Pelagic sea snakes are true ocean-going snakes, and may be seen hundreds of miles from land. They do reach the continental shelf of South America, including the Gulf of California.

Although sea snakes abound, and are poisonous, they are shy and because of this are usually harmless. There have been no know fatalities from sea snakes in the Americas.

CHAPTER FIVE

REPTILES

HISTORICAL VIEW OF SNAKES

SNAKES HOLD A UNIQUE POSITION in the animal world in the minds of men. From the earliest recorded history they have been venerated, deified, despised, and feared more than any other animal.

Ra, the sun god of Egyptian Mythology supposedly stepped on a snake while making earth. His case history, compiled around 1500 B.C. indicates the symptoms following cobra envenomation.

The cobra and cerastes appeared in the architecture, friezes, and writings of nearly every dynasty. The cobra was used as a symbol of vitality and benevolence in the royal crown of Egypt. The Egyptian idea of the universe included a serpent who cradled the earth in its coils to protect it. Paradise was guarded by fire-breathing snakes.

The underworld was thought to be ruled by a huge snake who battled with Ra each night, and each morning's light showed that Ra had triumphed again. An eclipse was viewed as a temporary event with the serpent holding sway. Snakebite victims were considered profaned and the eternal spirit would not live in them.

Ophiolatry in the surrounding countries was prevalent, although not related to Egyptian religion. Moses and Aaron were considered snake shamans by the Israelites, and indeed Moses had a bronze serpent made which was destroyed by Hezekiah. Python worship was common in Africa and this was brought to the West Indies where voodoo developed. Natives in Africa still believe their ancestors have been reincarnated as snakes.

European history also contains a plethora of snake fables. Many of the Greek gods and goddesses were part snake or descended from snakes. The early Druids used snakes in their rites. The Druids resisted St. Patrick when he tried to christianize Ireland, and he supposedly drove the snakes off in a fit of anger.

Northern European mythology is full of venomous snakes. Their version of hell was a dark cold place made of snakes bodies, with a constant flow of cold venom forming a river.

Snake worship no doubt reached a peak in India, and has persisted until modern times in many parts of the subcontinent. Buddhism abounds with snake myths, most of which picture the serpents in a benevolent light. They were given human characteristics and were supposedly converted by Buddha, although he felt they were inferior beings who were reincarnated as cobras because of some evil deed. The Hindus believe the serpent Shesha was important in creation. This snake was similar to that of the Buddhist's in that it was generally benevolent with many virtious qualities.

The snake myths of the New World are very similar to those elsewhere, with one slight change—the rattlesnake is the object of deification or humanization in the New World. Medicines were compounded from dried snake rattles, dried flesh, eyes, and so forth. Snakes were also credited with being able to control the weather, and bring good or bad luck. These myths were prevalent throughout North and South America.

The Shawnee Indians viewed thunder as the voice of a godly rattlesnake, and the Sioux believed lightning was a rattlesnake striking. The best known myth or practice is that of the Hopi Indians—each year they have a snake dance to insure rainfall and fertility.

Serpents figure prominently in our Judeo-Christian heritage. We are all familiar with the story of Adam and Eve in the Garden of Eden. Here the Serpent is pictured as the antithesis of God. There are approximately fifty references to serpents in the King James Bible and almost all of them picture the snake as evil.

The early settlers in America sent word back to Europe telling fabulous stories of the rattlesnakes. Snakes were very uncommon in Europe at that time and rattlesnakes seemed to captivate the imagination. The rattlesnake was adopted as a symbol for colonial America. The motto "Don't Tread on Me" was emblazoned on a banner with a coiled rattler. In view of these supernatural feelings, it is small wonder that snakebite was so feared on the early American frontier. Wood, the authority on snakes for many years, stated in 1855 that bites were always fatal, the victims dying usually within a few hours. Many other authors agreed with him, and it was a common misunderstanding on the frontier that snakebites were almost always fatal. This is absolutely not true, the mortality rate for untreated snakebites probably is 3-10 percent and for treated bites, under 1 percent. This means, of course, that about 90 percent of snakebite victims will survive with no treatment. In frontier times many valueless treatments, including gunpowder, raw chickens, mud, and tobacco, were used with no benefit, but the fact that the victim survived was used as evidence of the efficacy of the treatment.

GENERAL FACTS ABOUT SNAKES IN THE WESTERN HEMISPHERE

Snakes are found throughout the United States, Mexico, Central and South America, and in parts of Canada. They are cold-blooded (poikilothermic) animals, and their body temperature is that of the surrounding climate. This factor makes life for them much easier in a warm climate than in a cold one. However, they are unable to sweat or lower their body temperature. Reptiles accommodate for this inability by taking advantage of natural temperature differences—they come out in the sun on a cool day and crawl in a hole on a hot one. Since the ground surface temperatures in the desert in the daytime are high enough to kill a snake in a few minutes, desert-dwelling snakes spend their days covered with sand or in holes. They become active at night when the temperatures drop. Snakes in cooler sections of the country usually are active in the day with no adverse results.

Snakes are most alert and their bodily functions are optimal in temperatures ranging from 80°–90°F. They die when their body temperature reaches 116°F. Cold is not as fatal as heat, but snakes rapidly develop a torpor and are very inactive around 40°F. Reptiles usually will not survive freezing, although there are a few isolated reports of apparently frozen snakes surviving when gradually warmed up.

Snakes usually become inactive during winter except on an occasional very warm day. Rattlesnakes in the colder areas seek dens in which to spend the winter. The dens are below the frost line to prevent freezing and are dry. Also they are usually protected from the north wind. The snakes tend to return to their dens in the fall and leave in the spring. The dens will contain many snakes, from 40 up to several hundred. There have been isolated reports of snake dens with over 1000 snakes. As the weather gets progressively colder, the snakes in the den group themselves into masses or "balls" of snakes often as big as a washtub. This prevents heat loss. On a warm day in fall the snakes may leave the den to lie about its entrance. One may find several hundred snakes lying about the den entrance on a mild fall day. Snakes in the warmer climates do not tend to den up as much as their colleagues in the colder climates. They may winter in holes and under stumps, and often do so singly or in limited numbers.

The cold weather dens tend to be permanent. Homes inadvertently built next to a rattlesnake den are due to be plagued with large numbers of snakes. The problem will persist to some degree until the den is destroyed. Dens may be located by noting which way the snakes are traveling in the fall and by searching for a large number of snakes sunning themselves on warm days.

The majority of snakes are harmless and nonpoisonous. The nonpoisonous ones are beneficial to mankind and should not be killed. They not only eat rats, mice, and small vermin that destroy crops but also keep poisonous snakes away by reducing the food supply. In addition, king snakes, racers, black snakes, and indigo snakes will kill and eat poisonous snakes.

HOW TO TELL A POISONOUS SNAKE

The ability to tell a poisonous snake from a nonpoisonous one is very important. Size, configuration, presence or absence of pits, and so forth all have been advocated as a means of identifying snakes. However, the one thing that makes a poisonous snake poisonous is the ability to inject the poison into an animal. Fangs are necessary for this. A poisonous snake therefore *must possess fangs*, and conversely the *absence of fangs* indicates a nonpoisonous one. This is true worldwide.

All snakes have small teeth, and these should not be confused with fangs. The fangs are located on the upper jaw in front just beneath the nostrils. The fangs of the pit viper are hollow and movable and usually lie flat against the roof of the mouth. They are rotated into position for striking. Many other snakes, especially in other countries, have fixed fangs which are usually smaller but present nonetheless. Some snakes have short, fixed fangs, located

in the rear of the mouth. For all practical purposes, however, these snakes are harmless to man.

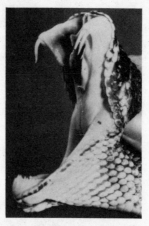

Pit Viper Fangs.
The eastern diamondback rattlesnake *(Crotalus adaman-
theus)* is typical. Note the large, fleshy attachment, into
which the fangs fold when not in use. Fangs are replaced
constantly, and a new one has grown in on one side before
the old one was lost.

SNAKEBITE PREVENTION

The adage "an ounce of prevention is worth a pound of
cure" is especially true in the cases of snakes. The easiest
way to avoid being bitten is simple: Do not put your
hands or feet where you cannot see!

In snake country observe the following:

1. When walking, keep your eye on your path and avoid
stepping into clumps of brush or weeds. If you must
walk through brush, poke the clumps ahead of you with
a stick to rouse any reptile that may be there. Snakes
ordinarily do not attack people, and they will be just
as happy for a chance to leave as you are for them to
leave.

2. Don't step over logs or large rocks if you cannot see over them. Step on the log first, then go over.

3. Wear heavy leather high-top shoes and loose fitting pants. Let the cuffs of the pants come down over the top of the shoes. Should a reptile attempt to strike, the pants will snag its fangs and very likely cause premature closing of the jaws.

4. Go under fences in cleared areas only.

5. Do not walk close to rock ledges.

6. Do not reach above your head and put your hand in crevices while climbing.

7. Do not move when you hear a snake rattle. Snakes usually strike at moving objects. If you back away from one snake, don't back into another.

8. Do not water ski where water moccasins are plentiful.

9. Sleeping on the ground is ill advised. Although snakes ordinarily do not attack, you may inadvertently roll over on one or put an arm or leg on one.

10. Remember, a favorite resting place for snakes is under discarded lumber, debris, and firewood. Wear heavy gloves when cleaning up material like this. Before picking up a discarded board, use a crowbar or piece of lumber to raise one end of the board so you can see if it is safe to pick it up. Do the same with firewood and kindling. Snakes also like to crawl under the floor of corncribs, abandoned barns and houses. Be careful when walking or working in them.

If you own a summer or vacation cottage, a few simple precautions will make it snakeproof.

1. Always ask about snakes before buying or building a cabin. Snakes may be plentiful in one area and completely absent in another right beside it.

2. Keep the grass, weeds, and brush cut so snakes cannot hide. Doing this should make it safe to walk to boat docks etc.

3. Keep debris cleaned up. Do not leave garbage where it will attract rats and mice, which are a principal food supply for snakes.

4. Do not kill nonpoisonous snakes! They keep the food supply depleted and keep the population of poisonous snakes down.

5. Never pick up an apparently dead snake. There may

be more life in it than you think. Experiments have shown that a snake head severed from its body will remain alive and able to inflict a deadly bite for 15–30 minutes after being severed. Should you feel it necessary to pick up a snake, use a stick and put the snake in a large sack, holding it away from your body.

For more detailed information on snakes and their habits the following books are suggested:

Rattlesnakes, Their Habits, Life Histories, and Influence on Mankind by L. M. Klauber, Berkeley: University of California Press, 1956.

Snakes of the World by Raymond L. Ditmars, New York: The Macmillan Company, 1931.

VENOMOUS SNAKES IN THE UNITED STATES

The dangerous snakes in the United States are all members of the Crotalidae, or pit viper family, or the Elapidae, or coral snake family. The pit vipers are movable-fanged snakes, and the coral snakes are fixed-fanged snakes.

There is a third type of snake which, although rare,

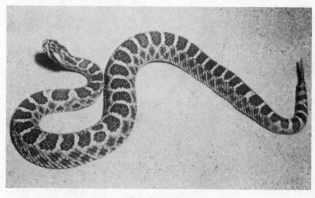

Rattlesnake.
Note the broad head, narrow neck, and rattles on the tail. Very variable in color.
PHOTOGRAPH COURTESY OF ROSS ALLEN REPTILE FARM, SILVER SPRINGS, FLORIDA.

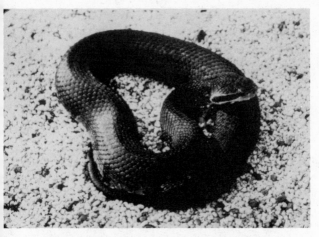

Water Moccasin (Ancistrodon piscivorous).
Fairly large—up to six feet—with a heavy body. The inside of the mouth is white, giving the snake the popular name of Cottonmouth. Olive, black, or brown, sometimes with dark crossbands on the back. Probably the most belligerent snake in North America. Bites are most frequent in the lower Mississippi valley and along the Gulf coast. Death is rare, but tissue destruction may be severe.

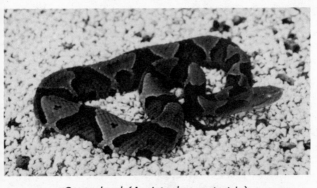

Copperhead (Ancistrodon contortrix).
About three feet long. The belly is white, and the head is copper or pink. There are brown crossbands or "hourglass" markings on the back, with the narrow part at the center of the back. These alternate with gray or light yellow bands.

should be mentioned. These are the rear-fanged snakes of the family Colubridae. They are venomous, but the short, fixed fangs are located so far posteriorly that a strike is impossible. One would have to put one's finger in the snake's mouth and let it chew on the finger to get envenomated. There is no record of any deaths or injuries from these snakes. Species of this type of snake include the Senora and California lyre snakes, found in southern California and Nevada; the Texas lyre snake, found in west Texas; and the Mexican vine snake, found in southern Arizona.

Pit Vipers

The pit vipers include the rattlesnakes, moccasins, and copperhead in the United States, the bushmaster in South America, the *Bothrops* in Mexico and South America, and the *Trimeresurus* in Asia. They are so named because they have a pit below the nostril. The pit is a heat-sensitive device that aids in directing the snake in striking its victim. Pit vipers are found in almost all the 48 continental states.

PATHOLOGY OF PIT VIPER VENOM

The venom produced by the pit viper is used for feeding rather than for defense. For self-protection these snakes rely on coloration and lack of natural enemies. The venom is a "prehensile" complex which secures, kills, and digests the prey. It is peculiar in that it is most effective against rodents, rabbits, frogs, and other animals that die almost immediately. The prey is ingested whole, and the injected venom completes the digestion. Envenomation in other animals is extremely varied.

The venom has been shown to be neurotoxic, hemorrhagic, thrombogenic, hemolytic, proteolytic, and antibactericidal. It has the same effects as antifibrin and anticoagulants have on the blood and ferments and kinases have in digestion (22). It contains four factors which are present in varying amounts in each species of pit vipers. These factors are: (a) neurotoxic, (b) spreading, (c) digestive, and (d) hemorrhagic. *Crotalus adamanteus* (eastern diamondback) venom has the highest concentration of the digestive factors (23). *Crotalus scutulatus scutulatus* (the Mojave rattlesnake) has the highest concentration of the neurotoxic factor (11).

In humans, digestive factor causes more morbidity than the neurotoxic factor. Local reaction or loss of limb is caused by digestion of muscle with resultant edema. This edema causes a marked increase in the subfascial tension, great enough to occlude arterial blood flow with subsequent gangrene of the extremity.

Systemic reaction to *Crotalus* envenomation is extremely variable, even with the same species of snake. Deaths have been reported from hemorrhage in the bowel and bladder or subcutaneous, intraperitoneal, and intrathoracic hemorrhage. In some reactions, neurotoxic features such as fasciculation, immediate, severe, generalized weakness, and painful cramps are dominant.

FIRST AID

One dictum every doctor learns in his first year of medical school is "First, do not harm." Unfortunately, many of the first aid measures recommended in the popular press and journals have yet to subscribe to this philosophy. Many of the treatments have very little value, and others are actually dangerous. A few sacred cows deserve to be slain here.

1. Cutting and sucking the wound. There is no argument with the fact that snake venom can be retrieved by immediate sucking on the wound (22, 39). Incisions, however, are a different story. Many bites are at the base of the thumb, and the recurrent branch of the median nerve may be cut while incising a fang mark. The ulnar nerve, on the other side of the hand, is also vulnerable. Perma-

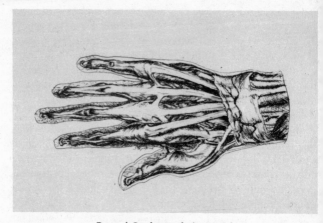

Dorsal Surface of the Hand.
The extensor tendons lie just beneath the skin and can easily be damaged by incision, resulting in inability to extend the fingers at the metacarpophalangeal joint.

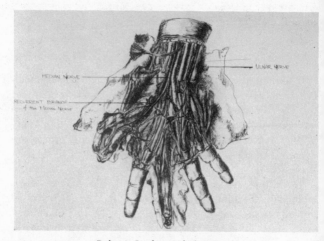

Palmar Surface of the Hand.
Many bites are on the hand. The radial and ulnar nerves lie just beneath the skin, making any incision on the palm or around the base of the thumb very dangerous.

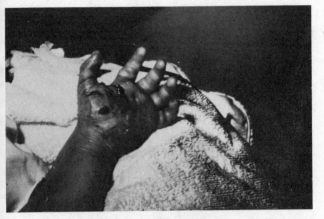

Fang Marks on the Thenar Eminence.
Any cutting on this hand by an inexperienced person could well injure the median nerve or its recurrent branch, resulting in loss of sensation and inability to oppose the thumb to the fingers.

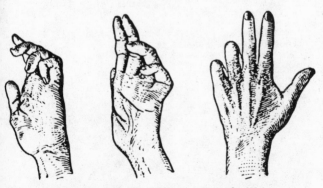

Result of Cutting the Ulnar Nerve at the Wrist.
This injury is often overlooked because most of the finger movements are apparently intact. The result, however, is an almost useless hand—far too high a price to pay for a careless incision.

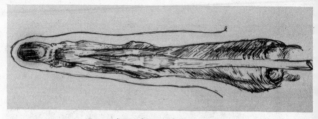

Dorsal Surface of the Finger.
The extensor mechanism lies just beneath the skin. Any incision in this area may result in finger drop.

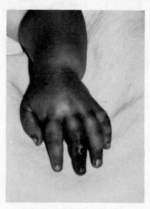

Rattlesnake Bite on the Back of the Middle Finger.
Incision of the fang marks here would be very dangerous because of the many tendons, nerves, and arteries in the small space.

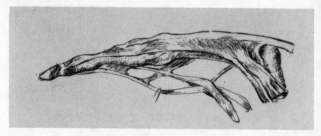

Lateral Surface of the Finger.
The complex, closely packed structures are easily damaged and difficult to repair, making any incision ill advised.

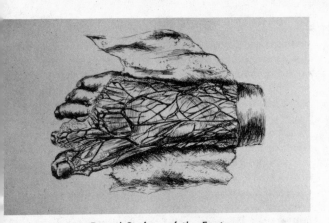

Dorsal Surface of the Foot.
The many tendons are important in dorsiflexion of the toes.
Although toe motions are not as important as finger motions,
loss of them is bad enough to be avoided scrupulously. If
incisions are done at all, it should be by a trained doctor.

nent paralysis of a hand may follow. Incisions on a hand
should be made only by doctors, *never* by enthusiastic
first-aiders. Do not use mouth suction. Instead, keep a
snakebite kit handy, with its rubber suction cup. Suction
should be started within 3 minutes and may be discon-
tinued in 15–30 minutes. It should be emphasized that
this is a *first aid* procedure and not primary therapy. Results are extremely variable and no time should be lost in
taking the victim to a hospital or doctor.

2. Tourniquets. Tourniquets should *not* be used in the
initial treatment of snake bite. They are dangerous! Ex-
perimentially, tourniquets have been found to have little
value (23). Using a tourniquet will not prevent death and
can cause extensive necrosis (11). Loosening the tourniquet may produce shock and death may follow (49).

3. Ice treatment or cryotherapy. This should not be
done by lay people. Damage to the limb may be made
worse (2, 22, 30, 50, 52), and an amputation may be
necessary.

4. Do not waste time hunting for the snake! Personal

reasons may prompt one to find the snake and kill it, but this should be done after the victim is on the way to the doctor or hospital. Please do not feel constrained to present the reptile remains to the doctor or hospital for viewing. First, the snake may not be dead and may recover at an inopportune moment. Second, few physicians are able to identify most snakes. Third, it makes no difference what kind of snake it is since only one pit viper antivenin is available. The amount needed depends on the severity of the injury and not on the kind of snake. There are two exceptions, however. The Mojave rattlesnake produces a primarily neurotoxic venom. Its victims require much more antivenom than is apparent from observation of the wound. And the coral snake produces a different type of neurotoxic venom, for which a separate antivenom is available.

So far attention has been focused first on what *not* to do rather than what to do because the *don'ts* are so much more important than the do's. But there are a few do's.

1. The first and foremost objective of first aid treatment for snakebite is to get the victim to a doctor or hospital as quickly as possible. However, a hair-raising dash through crowded intersections and red lights is absolutely not indicated. A safe, sane, calm drive in a car or truck is the best.

2. Keep the patient as quiet as possible. Splint the arm or leg with pillows, rolled up magazines or some other comfortable material—*not* rigid poles tied on with ropes. Do the best you can to keep general body activity, such as running, to an absolute minimum. Wild animals instinctively keep quiet when they are bitten, and there is good clinical evidence that this is beneficial (8, 11, 22, 34).

The most difficult task is to convince the trained first-aider that such a common and mundane thing as going to a doctor is the best treatment. The popular misconception persists that an immediate use of knives, tourniquets, ice, and serum, is all that stands between the patient and sudden death, and this is simply not true. Snakebites are an emergency, of course, but not an extreme one. There is no reason not to inspect the patient and develop a logical plan of treatment. As in other reactions, the presence of denatured protein and blood in the extremity secondary to protein digestion, leads to shock, renal and hepatic shutdown, and myocardial failure.

Although more people in the world die from snakebite than all other animal bites combined (49), in the United States loss of limbs, rather than death, is the usual criterion of unsuccessful treatment. Ninety-eight percent of the bites are on the extremities (52). Limb loss seems to be more common in children, who seem to be more sensitive to snake venom than adults. Seventeen percent of post-traumatic amputations in children under 15 under the care of the Florida Crippled Children's Commission were the result of venomous snake bites. (21)

DEFINITIVE TREATMENT

The initial steps in the definitive treatment of snakebite are:

1. Look for fang marks. All poisonous snakes have fangs, and no harmless ones have them. Therefore, no fang marks, no envenomation (19). All snakes have small teeth that may make a scratch or laceration. These are easily distinguished from fang marks on close examination. Remember that only one fang may have penetrated.

2. Assess the severity of the bite. Fundamental to the treatment of any disease is an estimate of the severity of the disease. The treatment of snakebite is no different. Fortunately about 30 percent of all snakebites give no evidence of envenomation. These cases require observation only. Pain and swelling are the two chief results of envenomation that are immediately observed. An estimate of the degree of pain and swelling will indicate the amount of venom present. Wood, Hoback, and Green established three grades of envenomation (51). Parrish added Grade 0 for patients who were fanged but not envenomated (28). Gennaro later added Grade IV to include severe bites of the large rattlesnakes.

The estimated number of vials of antivenin required for each grade is listed in Table 2. Examination of the fang marks should enable one to tell rather quickly the approximate grade of envenomation. Frequent reexamination will be necessary during the first few hours. One should of course not wait 10–12 hours to definitely establish the degree of envenomation before starting the administration of antivenin. Remember, children require more antivenin than adults.

3. Start an I.V. in the contralateral arm with a needle large enough to administer blood. Draw enough blood at

Table 2. Grades and Treatment of Envenomation Severity

Severity		Number of Vials of Antivenin
0.	Fang marks—no envenomation: Reveals 1″ wheal or less in the first 12 hours	0
I.	Mild envenomation:	1-2
II.	Moderate envenomation: Severe pain, tenderness, edema extending 10″-15″ within 12 hours, erythema, petechiae, ecchymosis, weakness, nausea, vomiting, bloody ooze at the fang marks	2-5 Moderate (86% of all bites) Severe (14% of all bites)
III.	Severe envenomation: Widespread pain, tenderness, edema extending 10″-20″ within 12 hours, petechiae, ecchymosis, weakness, nausea, vertigo and vomiting appearing rapidly	5-10
IV.	Very severe envenomation: Rapid swelling, may affect ipsilateral trunk, ecchymosis, bleb formation, weakness, vertigo, vomiting, hematemesis, tingling about face and head, fasciculation, muscle cramping, possible paralysis, yellow vision, blindness, shock, convulsions	10-30

Source: Wood, J. T., Haback, W. W., and Green, T. W. "Treatment of snake venom poisoning with ACTH and cortisone." *Virginia Medical Monthly* 82 (1955): 130–35. Rep. 51.

the same time for a complete blood count and a type and cross match. Often blood transfusions are required and if the physician delays too long in obtaining a specimen for typing and cross matching, it may be impossible to cross match the blood. Have blood available.

4. Skin test for antivenin sensitivity. This could be done while the I.V. is being started.

MODERATE ENVENOMATION: GRADE I, II

In cases of mild to moderate envenomation, hemolysis and/or a very severe bleeding diathesis may be a part of the picture, and there may be severe depletions of fibrinogen and platelets and large fluid losses. Transfusions of whole blood (preferably fresh), plasma, and platelets may be necessary. Renal shutdown may require dialyses.

For mild to moderate envenomation, continue treatment as follows.

5. Add the appropriate amount of antivenin to the I.V. fluids which have already been started. The I.V. should be running at a rate to deliver the antivenin in 3 to 4 hours. *Do not* give the antivenin intramuscularly. Desensitization may be necessary prior to giving the antivenin if the skin test is positive.

6. Start the patient on broad spectrum antibiotics.

7. Give tetanus prophylaxis.

8. Enlarge the fang marks by making 2 mm. incisions transversely at either side of fang marks.

9. Control pain. This can very simply be done in this case with meperidine (Demerol) or morphine.

10. Do not permit the patient to take any food or liquids by mouth.

11. Check the circulation distal to the bite at least every hour. This is very important. The increase in subfascial tension may occlude arterial flow and subsequent gangrene of the extremity distal to the bite may occur.

The tissue destruction after a snakebite results in marked edema. If the fangs are large enough to give a deeper envenomation, an appreciable amount of subfascial edema may ensue. This results in a relative compromise of the circulation distal to the bite. Therefore, it is mandatory that the circulation distal to the bite be checked *at least every hour.* Relaxation incisions in the deep fascia may be necessary to save the function of the extremity.

One recommended method of fasciotomy is to make several transverse incisions in the skin approximately 1″ long and 3″ apart. The dissection is carried to the deep fascia which is incised in a longitudinal manner. This results in multiple skin "bridges" which permit the release of tension but keep the muscles and so forth from herniating out. An escape of serosanguineous fluid ensues, further reducing pressure. A successful fasciotomy shows marked and immediate improvement in the distal tissues. General improvement is also noted.

Fasciotomy may be done by simply splitting the skin and fascia with a longitudinal incision. Although this is quick and effective, some tissue may extravasate and slough later, and the scar is more unsightly. Glass combined fasciotomy with excision of the bite area and achieved good results (12).

12. Check vital signs hourly and urine for blood every hour. Check blood count every 4 hours for evidence of hidden bleeding or hemolysis.

SEVERE ENVENOMATION: GRADE III OR IV

In treating cases of severe envenomation, the initial four steps (pp. 55–57) remain the same. The following regimen is then used.

5. Add the appropriate amount of antivenin to the I.V. and run it in in 3 or 4 hours. The quicker the antivenin can be gotten to the venom the better. When the venom is neutralized (the United States Public Health Service states that 1 cc. of the antivenin will neutralize 1.75 mg. of venom), the signs and symptoms of envenomation will regress.

6. Excise the bite if patient is seen within an hour of being bitten. Experiments with tagged venom have shown that 50 percent of venom can be removed by excision if it is done before one hour passes (41). In the case of severe envenomation, the bite should excised even if it has been over an hour since the victim was bitten.

Debridement of the bite is carried out in the operating room with the patient under anesthesia (regional block such as axillary for the upper extremity or spinal for the lower extremity is satisfactory). All necrotic tissue is excised at this time. Edema of the underlying muscle compartment will indicate the need for a fasciotomy. At the same time, good hemostas is obtained and the skin is left open. Several days later the skin may be closed or skin grafts done.

7. Use axillary block or spinal anesthesia for relief of pain. This has the added advantage of blocking the sympathetic nervous system and increasing blood supply to the extremity.

8. A tourniquet may be used above the edematous area *only* if it appears that a *catastrophy* is imminent. Recent experiments have shown that the venom incarcerated in the extremity may do more damage to the extremity (50). Also, deaths have been reported when the tourniquet is removed and a large bolus of digested protein, blood, and venom is suddenly released in the systemic circulation.

The antivenin should be circulating at least 30–60 minutes before the tourniquet is removed. The extremity distal to the tourniquet should be drained of as much blood as possible with a needle in the vein. The tourniquet should occlude the venous return but not arterial supply—thus a crude perfusion is possible. *Use of a tourniquet may aid in saving a life, but only with concomitant increase in danger to the limb.*

9. Check distal circulation. If the arterial circulation becomes occluded (usually at the wrist and ankles), fasciotomy may be necessary. Transverse incisions should be made in the skin and vertical incisions in the fascia. This

relieves the pressure, and has sort of a gridiron effect to keep the muscles from herniating through and sloughing. Incisions in the same plane are contraindicated since the subfascial pressure is so great that there will be a large extravasation of muscle and tissue with subsequent loss. However, incisions in the same plane may be necessary in *very severe* cases. In these cases the extremity is simply cut open from one end to the other. Grafts may be needed later.

10. Maintain blood pressure and pulse, insert a Foley catheter and check the urine for volume and blood. Be prepared to maintain respiration and blood volume.

11. Give tetanus prophylaxis and broad spectrum antibiotics.

The July 1971 issue of *Hospital Medicine* reports on the results of using fasciotomy and steroids in 9 cases of severe envenomation by rattlesnakes. All the gangrenous tissues, blebs, and blisters were debrided. Fasciotomies were then done to release the subfascial tension. Large amounts of fluid were noticed extruding. Intravenous fluids and blood were administered as needed, monitored if necessary by central venous pressure. Generalized symptoms, nausea, vomiting, and shock were treated with intravenous fluids and 1 gm. of hydrocortisone sodium succinate given intravenously every 4–6 hours as needed for as long as 72 hours.

This form of treatment is valueless in the case of neurotoxic venoms.

ANTIVENIN

Antivenin is the keystone of successful snakebite treatment. Pit viper antivenin is manufactured from hyperimmune horse serum. The venoms used for its manufacture are from the tropical rattler (*C. d. terrificus*), the fer-de-lance (*Bothrops atrox*), the eastern diamondback, (*C. adamanteus*) and the western diamondback (*C. atrox*). The antivenin is effective against all North and South American pit vipers, those of Korea and Japan, and the

Trimeresurus species of the Pacific Islands. It is available at most hospital emergency rooms and larger drug stores.

Antivenin made from goat antiserum and human antiserum is available only at U.C.L.A. This is made from *C. atrox* (western diamondback) and is not commercially available at the present time.

REACTIONS TO ANTIVENIN

The immediate reaction to antivenin is similar to that of horse serum anaphylaxis. To treat these reactions, simply shut off the I.V. flow and administer adrenalin through the I.V. tubing. It is suggested that a syringe of adrenalin be kept loaded and available when administering the horse serum intravenously.

Serum sickness may occur in 6 to 24 days. Symptoms are fever, malaise, lymphadenopathy, arthralgia, and urticaria. Neurological signs such as meningismus or peripheral neuritis may occur. The peripheral neuritis usually involves the shoulders and arms (upper brachial plexus). Pain and muscle weakness are frequently present and permanent atrophy may develop. Cortisone is beneficial for these conditions. Accelerated reactions are the same but occur in a few minutes to 2 to 5 days.

Local reactions are usually manifested by progressive erythema (rash), edema, and itching of the skin-tested area. The Arthus phenomenon occurs at the site of repeated injections. There is local necrosis which may progress to gangrene and slough. This is avoided by giving the antivenin intravenously during the initial 24-hour period of administration.

ANTIVENIN SENSITIVITY

The most common question physicians ask is "What do I do in the case of antivenin sensitivity?" The introduction of horse serum products in an allergic individual is very dangerous and may cause death. Severe snakebites, on the other hand, will cause death unless the antivenin is administered.

In the case of pit viper envenomation, it is well to remember that 30 percent of all bites have no envenomation and consequently no antivenin is needed. In an additional 56 percent envenomation is mild to moderate and probably could be treated adequately by supportive measures. This leaves about 14 percent of pit viper bites requiring antivenin. The classical treatment for antivenin hyperallergy is desensitization. Prepare a 1:100 solution of antiserum and inject 0.1, 0.2, and 0.5 cc. of the solution in the I.V. at 15 minute intervals. Then repeat with a 1:10 solution. A 1:1000 solution of epinephrine must be kept ready in a syringe to inject in the I.V. tubing as needed. In a real emergency, epinephrine may be injected into the I.V. prior to administering the antiserum.

ANTIVENIN INFUSION AND PERFUSION

Intra-arterial antivenin infusion and isolation perfusion techniques should be mentioned here. Although it is very unlikely that it would be necessary to use these techniques in this country, they are available and can be used in a catastrophic event. Snyder reported on cases in which he used arterial infusion of antivenin (41). For bites on the head he infused the antivenin into the carotid artery and for bites on the extremity, the femoral artery and brachial arteries. Unfortunately, he did not grade the bites so it is impossible to tell how severe the envenomation was. The procedure was simple. He added antivenin to I.V. fluids and pumped them into the artery using a needle and a regular bulb pump.

Experimental work on dogs indicates that an isolation perfusion system, in which an occlusive tourniquet is used above the bite and the antivenin is pumped into the artery and the appropriate vein drained, is probably the most effective treatment. However, although extremely good results have been obtained with dogs (19), I can find no instances where it has been used on human beings. This

treatment is fairly difficult and extreme and would probably be of more value in South America and Africa, where
the snakes are larger and envenomation more severe.

ANTIHISTAMINES AND CORTISONE

Do not use antihistamines. They have a synergistic
action with the venom and are contraindicated. Do not
use cortisone, as it evidently interferes with the antigen-
antibody reaction between the venom and antivenin.

ALCOHOL

Alcohol became popular as a snakebite remedy about
the 1850s. It was embraced not only by laymen but also
by eminent physicians. Many case reports were published
showing the benefits of alcohol. Alcohol was believed to
be a specific antidote for snakebite. It supposedly would
seek out venom in the body and neutralize it. It was felt
that anyone who had snakebite symptoms was merely
insufficiently supplied with alcohol, and that if one was
careful to take the precaution to drink a goodly amount
of alcohol prior to being bitten, he would be immune to
the venom. The volume of alcohol prescribed was enor-
mous. It was common to give from one ounce to one-half
pint of whisky every few minutes until the patient was
inebriated. Often one and one-half quarts were imbibed
in a day.

A reverse twist on this was the advocation of some physicians to use snake venom to cure alcoholism.

The introduction of antivenin in 1920 almost completely
eliminated the use of alcohol for snakebite. The physio-
logical action of the alcohol tends to spread the venom
and thus is contraindicated.

INCISION AND SUCTION

I am mentioning incision and suction separately because
it is a widely used procedure. The fang marks should be

enlarged about 2–3 mm. on each side and constant (not mouth) suction applied. If suction is started within 30 minutes of being bitten and the bite is subcutaneous, about 50 percent of the venom can be removed in this manner. However, suctioning a bite after 30 minutes has elapsed is valueless. Valuable time should not be lost in making incisions and starting suction as a first aid measure. A bad situation may become a desperate one in a short time. Vital structures, such as the ulnar and median nerves, may inadvertently be damaged, and having to withstand the incision of an unanesthetized painful wound by an inexperienced person may make the patient nervous and hyperactive and enhance the spread of the venom.

Incision and suction done in a hospital setting by a physician is a safe procedure, but as mentioned, unless it is done within 30 minutes of being bitten, it is ineffective. It probably is not necessary in cases of mild envenomation and may be beneficial in cases of moderate (grade II) envenomation, but in severe envenomation, excision of the bite is much more effective. At best suction is an adjunct of definitive treatment, *not* a fundamental procedure.

Interestingly, although it has been proved in the laboratory that venom can be retrieved by cutting and sucking, there is no clinical work proving that it is advantageous in human envenomation. This seems strange until one realizes that most snakebites occur in situations where no medical personnel are available, and most lay people are reluctant to start cutting and sucking. Usually by the time a physician sees the patient, too much time has elapsed for the procedure to be of any use.

CRYOTHERAPY

A popular treatment for snakebite that was advocated recently is cryotherapy. The procedure and the theory behind it was simple and beguiling. A ligature was applied above the bite to keep the venom from spreading, and then the envenomated extremity was immersed in ice.

Cooling the extremity retarded the action of the venom, and there was no apparent tissue damage. The tourniquet was then removed and the venom was absorbed by the body. After a nonspecific period of time the extremity was warmed and the danger supposedly passed. The advantages of this treatment were immediately obvious. There was no need to use antivenin with its danger of adverse reactions. The patients usually looked and felt fairly well. However, the warming up of the envenomated extremity demonstrated the fallacy of this type of treatment. The limbs rapidly showed extensive necrosis. Many series reported showed beyond a shadow of a doubt that the use of cryotherapy markedly increased the incidence of amputations, sloughs, and necrosis.

Although the literature of the past few years has been practically unanimous in condemning this form of treat-

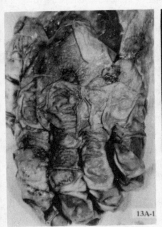 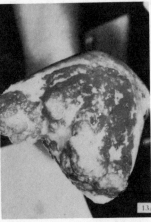

Macerated Hand.
The photograph on the left shows a hand that was immersed in ice water for more than forty-eight hours. The photograph on the right shows the same hand after removal of all dead tissue.

PHOTOGRAPHS COURTESY OF NEWTON MC CULLOUGH, TUBAC, ARIZONA. PUBLISHED FIRST IN THE FLORIDA STATE MEDICAL JOURNAL.

ment, unfortunately it is still being used with many sloughs and malpractice suits following (4, 36, 42). There is one situation, however, in which cryotherapy could be used beneficially and that is in cases where amputation is a foregone conclusion. In such cases, it could be used to gain time needed for preoperative preparation of the patient, or it could be used when it is evident that the amputation cannot be carried out for a long time. In any event, this should be explained to the patient and his permission for the amputation obtained before beginning treatment.

COMMON ERRORS IN TREATMENT

The most common errors in treating snakebites are:

1. Using insufficient amounts of antivenin. Careful scrutiny of charts of fatal cases reveal a reluctance on the part of physicians to administer adequate amounts of antivenin. Fifteen to 30 vials should be administered. At least half of the antinvenin should be given in the first few hours and the rest of it within the first 24 hours.

2. Administering the antivenin intramuscularly instead of intravenously. Reports in fatal cases often indicate that the antivenin was given intramuscularly or subcutaneously because the physicians were reluctant to give large amounts of horse serum intravenously. Studies using tagged antivenin have shown that 84.9 percent of the antivenin is localized at the site of envenomation 2 hours after intravenous administration. In contrast, only 1.43 percent is found at the site 2 hours after intramuscular administration and 5.6 percent after subcapular administration (50).

Coral Snakes

Coral snakes belong the the Elapidae family, which also includes the cobras, kraits, and mambas. In the Western Hemisphere, coral snakes are all found in tropical or sub-

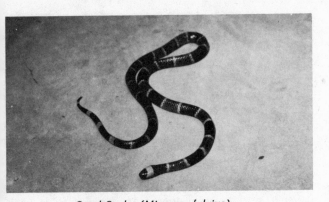

Coral Snake (Micrurus fulvius).
Note the slender body and small bullet head. The eyes are small, with round pupils. The body appears waxy and has rings of black, red, and yellow. The head is usually black. In the North American variety (but not the tropical varieties), the red and yellow rings touch, and the red and black rings do not.

tropical climates and probably migrated from Asia. Three kinds are found in the United States. The eastern coral snake, *Micrurus fulvius fulvius*, is found in Florida, Georgia, Alabama, South Carolina, and North Carolina. This species is claimed to be found as far north as Tennessee and Kentucky. The Texas coral, *M. f. tenere*, is found in southwest Arkansas, Louisiana, Texas, and Mexico. The Arizona (or Sonora) coral, *M. euryxanthus*, is found in Arizona and New Mexico. It is small, secretive, and usually inoffensive.

Characteristically, the coral snake is a small thin snake with a small round black eye. Its fangs are fixed, not hollow, and the venom flows down grooves in the fangs. These snakes do not "strike" but hold and "chew" their victim. This allows the venom to flow over the wound into the fang marks. The snakes are waxy, shiny in appearance, and usually have alternating red, yellow, and black bands on their bodies and a black head. A black or melanistic form and a white albino form have been described. The coral snake lives under loose soil, leaves, and debris. It is a burrowing type of snake and is usually uncovered by

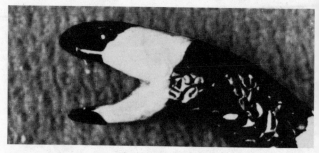

Coral Snake Fangs.
The short, fixed fangs are barely visible in the upper jaw.

raking or working in the ground. These snakes are shy and elusive, but when excited, their movements become rapid and apparently purposeless. However, these thrashing movements are designed to bring the snake's head close to the victim's body for the bite (22).

For the decade 1960–1969, only one death from a coral snake bite was reported. An antivenin is available, but it is not effective for the Arizona coral. But then there has never been a report of a death from this snake.

SYMPTOMS

Coral snake venom is almost purely paralytic in action. There is no tissue reaction and the pain is only that of the fangs. Symptoms usually do not appear for several hours. This is a characteristic of the coral and the krait bite, and initially it may lull the physician into a false sense of security. Several hours after the bite, apprehension, giddiness, ptosis of the eyelids, euphoria, lethargy, nausea, salivation, vomiting, and weakness occur. Convulsions may occur, along with a bulbar type paralysis, involving the cranial nerves, and respiratory paralysis. Peripheral paralysis follows, but the sensorium remains clear until death. All these effects of the venom apparently are reversible, and completely paralyzed patients have recovered.

If young children develop these signs unexpectedly while in the southern states, remember to check for fang marks. There have been instances where children either are not able to talk, or afraid to talk, and these signs of neuromuscular collapse have been due to the coral snake. Diagnosis in these instances was made by finding fang marks.

TREATMENT

All patients should be hospitalized.

1. Observe for symptoms of envenomation for at least 24 hours. Include respiration checks every 30 minutes.

2. Have a tracheostomy set, respirator, and antivenin available.

3. Check urine for blood every hour, since hematuria is a common finding.

4. Wash the bite area. Frequently there is venom deposited on the skin around the fang marks. Any attempt to cut and suck may reenvenomate the patient.

5. If signs of envenomation occur, start an I.V. with three to five vials of coral snake antivenin after skin testing. *Do not* give intramuscularly.

6. Give tetanus prophylaxis.

7. Do not use respiratory depressants. Use sedatives with extreme caution.

8. Maintain ventilation and blood pressure at all times.

ANTIVENIN

Coral snake antivenin is manufactured from horse serum using venom from *M. f. fulvius* (north Florida coral). It is effective against all coral bites except the Sonora coral snakes. This antivenin is available from the National Communicable Disease Center of the United States Public Health Service in Atlanta, Georgia (telephone 404-633-3311, or in emergencies, 404-633-2176). Many hospitals and poison control centers and state health departments of the southern states also stock the coral antivenin.

For information on reactions to antivenin and antivenin sensitivity see pp. 61–62.

Venomous Snakes in Other Countries of the Western Hemisphere

CANADA

A few species of rattlesnake are found in Canada. These species are also found in the United States and present no special problems.

MEXICO

The poisonous snakes of northern Mexico southward to Mexico City resemble those of the United States. However, approaching the tropical coastal plain the snake fauna rapidly changes.

Many coral snakes are found in Mexico, and they are very similar to those of the United States. They are highly venomous, but they are secretive and seldom encountered. In general, these snakes pose no serious threat. Most bites result from trying to catch the snake. Their venom is almost purely paralytic and produces almost no local tissue destruction. A polyvalent coral snake antivenin produced by the Instituto Butantan in Brazil is available.

The pit vipers are the most dangerous snakes in Mexico. These include the rattlesnakes of northern Mexico, which are similar to those of the southern United States, and the rattleless vipers of the New World, which include the genus *Bothrops*. Members of this genus are large (6–8 ft.) and very dangerous. They begin to be prominent in southern Mexico. A representative of the genus is the *Bothrops atrox*. These large brown or green-gray snakes are common in forests and along streams, and are often found in the plantations. The common name for this snake is the barba amarilla. Sometimes incorrectly called the fer-de-lance, it is probably the most dangerous snake and causes more deaths than any other snake in America. The pharmacological action of its venom is similar to that of the rattlesnakes. Treatment is the same as that advised for the larger rattlesnakes, but, due to the severity of the bite, a greater amount of antivenin will be necessary. The Wyeth polyvalent antivenin is effective as well as the antivenins produced by the Instituto Butantan in Brazil and the Laboratories Behrens in Venezuela.

Moving further south in Mexico, the deadly cascabel (*Crotalus durissis durissis*) is encountered. This is a fairly large rattlesnake found from southern Mexico to Central America. Its venom is different from that of most pit vipers in that the neurotoxic factor predominates. The clinical signs of envenomation are an early respiratory failure and a later paralysis. Blindness is also a common finding, and, indeed, "blindness and broken neck" are well known to physicians of Central and South America. The venom has only a limited local effect. This may lull the physician into a false sense of security at first for there is very little pain or swelling. The criteria given in Table 2 (p. 56) for determining the amount of antivenin needed are not valid

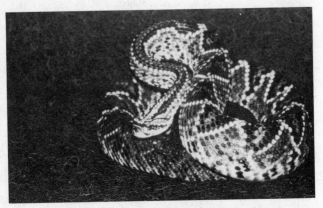

Cascabel (Tropical Rattlesnake) (Crotalus durissus terrificus).
Olive or brown, with yellow stripes on the neck, usually extending back only a few inches, but sometimes as much as 1/5 the length of the snake. Light belly and dark rhomboids edged with yellow on the back. Rhomboids are wider on the back than on the sides.
PHOTOGRAPH COURTESY OF TONY WILSON, GEORGETOWN, INDIANA.

for the cascabel. Anyone bitten by a cascabel should receive 10 ampules of antivenin as an initial dose, with possibly 20 or 30 being required (39).

Many other species of pit viper are found in Mexico, and many of them have rattles. However, these are either not important medically or they are so similar to the North American snakes that it would be repetitious to describe all of them.

CENTRAL AND SOUTH AMERICA

The southern Central American countries and northern South America give us the bushmaster (*Lachesis mutus*). This rattleless snake is the largest pit viper, attaining a length of 9–12 feet. It is a very formidable appearing snake with fangs averaging 1 inch. (Some have been found to be 1⅜ inches long.) This snake is potentially very dangerous because it secretes large amounts of venom. Few bites are recorded, however, probably due to the fact that it is strictly nocturnal and lives in abandoned burrows of mammals. A specific antivenin is produced by the Instituto Butantan in Brazil.

Many of the previously mentioned snakes are found in South America. The coral snakes are again present but, because of their habits, are only a minor hazard to life. However, their bite is serious since their venom is highly toxic, and a death rate approaching 50 percent has been reported. The venom has a marked neurotoxic effect and should be treated with antivenin. A polyvalent coral snake antivenin is produced by the Instituto Butantan in Brazil. Antivenin is also produced by the same institution for the northern coral snake (*M. frontalis*) and *M. corallinus*.

Although pit vipers are numerous, only one rattlesnake is found, the cascabel or *Crotalus durissis terrificus*. Although similar to the *C. d. durissis* of Mexico, the venom of the South American rattler apparently is more potent. This snake is responsible for more deaths than any other in Brazil. The venom is neurotoxic and insidious in action.

Rapid treatment with antivenin (probably 10–20 vials given intravenously) is mandatory. The grades of envenomation and amounts of antivenin advocated for other rattlesnake bites are not valid in this case.

Species of the *Bothrops* genus found in South America include the barba amarilla (*B. atrox*), the fer-de-lance (*B. lanceolatus*) the jararaca (*B. jararaca*), the jararacussu (*B. jararacussu*), and the Waglers pit viper (*B. neuwiedi*). The fer-de-lance is relatively unimportant and is found only on Martinique. The jararaca, a blotched, green-brown viper 3–4 feet long, is found in the central grasslands of South America. A very common snake, it is second to the cascabel in number of deaths it causes. It is not particularly venomous, and its victims should respond to antivenin and supportive treatment. The jararacussu is an aquatic

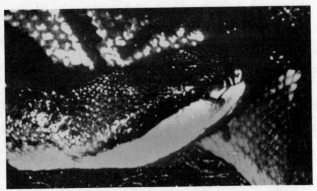

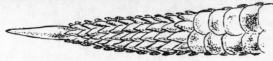

Bushmaster (Lachesis muta).
The largest of the pit vipers—up to 12 feet long. Rough skin. Tan to pale reddish brown with dark brown or black diamond-shaped blotches that are wide on the back and narrow on the sides. The rattle is absent, and a burr of pointed spines near the end of the tail is distinctive.

cousin of the *B. jajaraca*, but it is quite opposite. It is relatively uncommon, but has large amounts of a very toxic venom, making it one of the top four killers in South America. One of the early symptoms of envenomation is blindness, and early treatment with antivenin is indicated. The antivenin is available from Instituto Butantan in Brazil and Instituto Nacional de Microbiologia of Argentina. Waglers pit viper is a very common snake and probably causes more bites than any other snake, but relatively few deaths from it have been reported.

TREATMENT SUMMARY

The general principles of treatment are the same as for North American pit viper envenomation. Rest, supportive care, debridement, fasciotomy, administering antivenin, blood, and fluids, should be dispensed with a grain of clinical judgment. Bites from the neurotoxic pit vipers (the cascabel) must be treated whether symptoms have occurred or not. Remember, local signs of envenomation such as pain and swelling will not occur. The coral snakes of course are more common, larger, and more dangerous in tropical countries than the United States, but their secretive habits make them fairly unimportant as a cause of death. However, antivenins are available.

Imported Poisonous Snakes

There is a growing trend toward keeping imported poisonous reptiles in the home as a hobby. The Indian cobra is the most popular, but many other exotic, extremely poisonous, and frequently lethal snakes are being kept. This is a very dangerous practice and should not be done, because few physicians or hospital staffs in the United States have experience in treating these bites. Fortunately, there have been few accidents to date, but there are instances of the snakes escaping and biting their keepers or visitors. Luckily, foreign snakes do not live long in this climate.

Although there are no regulations governing the practice, a few rules should be followed if one decides to keep these snakes for there is the inevitable danger of being bitten or of the snake's escaping in populous areas.

1. The cages must be sound and locked at all times. Wire screening used for ventilation should be in two layers with an inch dead space between the layers so the snake cannot strike through the wire.

2. The cages must be durable enough so they will not open or break if they fall or someone knocks them over.

3. Snakes should not be taken out and exhibited to other people. They should not be let loose in a yard or place where they may escape.

4. Another person should be present when the snake is being fed or cleaned so that in case of an accident the victim could be taken to the hospital.

5. The keeper should know the scientific name and common name of any reptile he keeps.

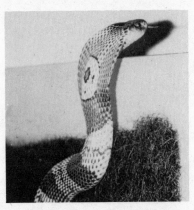

Indian Cobra (Naja naja).
Adults are brown or black, with a light belly, a black band on the lower neck, and a hood with a "spectacle" on the back. The markings are not visible in the black varieties.
PHOTOGRAPH COURTESY OF TONY WILSON, GEORGETOWN, INDIANA.

6. The keeper should keep or know where a supply of the oppropriate antivenin is located. It should be readily available, not across the country.

7. Should a snake escape, notify the local police and medical society. Include a description of the snake and the common and scientific name.

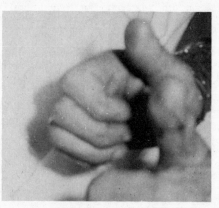

Cobra Bite on Thumb.
Cobra venom is completely neurotoxic and causes no swelling or tissue destruction.

TREATMENT

In case of snake bite do the following:

1. Capture the snake. It is imperative that the snake be identified.

2. Go to the hospital at once! A large teaching hospital would be preferable to a small community one in this instance because a respirator may be needed if the paralysis is rapid. Do not waste time with any first aid measures. Most of these venoms are neurotoxic and these procedures are largely valueless.

3. Examine for fang marks.

4. Obtain the antivenin as quickly as possible and administer it intravenously. The antivenin centers will send the correct amount.

5. Do not use cortisone, antihistamines, tourniquets,

ice, or incision and suction. These have no value and may do harm.

6. Take the usual precautions for treating a puncture wound. Wash the fang marks and give tetanus prophylaxis.

It must be emphasized that successful treatment of a victim of one of these foreign snakes is dependent on rapid intravenous administration of antivenin. Unfortunately, these antivenins can be very difficult to locate, especially late at night, on holidays, or on weekends. An inventory of foreign snake antivenins and information on where they can be obtained is given in the appendix.

Gila Monster

The Gila monster (*Heloderma suspectum*) and the basically similar Mexican beaded lizard (*Heloderma horridum*) are the only poisonous lizards in the world. The Mexican beaded lizard is found only in Mexico. The Gila monster is found in Arizona, southwestern Utah, New Mexico, and Sonora. It is chiefly a desert animal, sluggish, slow, timid, and retiring. It feeds on eggs, small birds, and mammals. Its teeth are short and grooved and break easily. Poison glands are located on the lower jaw. The lizard drools profusely when excited, opening and closing its mouth, bathing all its teeth in venom.

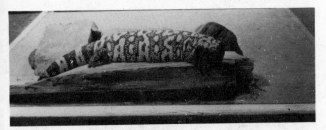

Gila Monster (Heloderma suspectum).
Note the heavy body and tail, short legs, and beaded appearance. Length about twenty inches.

There have been no deaths from Gila monster bites reported in the years 1960–1969. The only recorded death from 1929–1969 occurred in April 1930 (20). The victim was a 60-year-old man in Casa Grande, Arizona who died two hours after having been bitten. No hospital record is available but witnesses reported that he had been under the influence of alcohol and had received morphine.

The lizard's initial bite is marked by a tenacious grip and a side to side motion of its lower jaw. The animal may try to turn over on his back if irritated enough.

FIRST AID

First, get the victim loose from the animal quickly. It tends to clamp down for 5–10 minutes and the sooner it is disengaged, the less venom will be absorbed (20). Pry the jaws apart with a chisel, or strong tool if readily available. However, do not waste valuable time scouring the neighborhood for something to use. The alternative is so simple—pull the lizard off!! The teeth fortunately are easily pulled out and by simply grasping the lizard behind the forelegs it can easily be removed (20). Many other schemes have been suggested for ridding oneself of an unwanted Gila monster, but these should be avoided.

Second, get a doctor or go to a hospital. Severe bleeding has been reported and a pressure dressing may hastily be applied to control hemorrhage.

CLINICAL FINDINGS

The following symptoms have been observed: edema (may be due to the action of the teeth), severe pain, cyanosis around the wound, faintness, diaphoresis (profuse perspiration), nausea and vomiting, dyspnea (shortness of breath), slight paralysis, tachycardia, pallor, lymphangitis, "bulging" eyes, numbness, and seeing blinding lights. It will be noted that many of these symptoms are fairly general in nature and may be expected in any traumatic experience.

Since Gila monster wounds tend to bleed freely, the venom was thought to contain an anticoagulant. However, experimental work has not confirmed this. It seems likely that the bleeding is caused by the triangular teeth and the side to side crunching of the lizard's jaws when holding a victim. No generalized bleeding diathesis has been described.

Marked arteriospasm has been noted and probably accounts for the pain and cyanosis.

TREATMENT

1. Reassure the patient. Lowe and Limbacker state that death is not due solely to a Gila monster bite (13). The few deaths reported have been complicated by alcoholism and debility.

2. Administer broad spectrum antibiotics to control secondary infection.

3. Give tetanus prophylaxis.

4. If there is copious bleeding, simply irrigate the wound with normal saline and apply a dressing. If there is no bleeding, enlarge the puncture wounds slightly under local anesthesia.

5. Avoid cryotherapy and ligature. Although this procedure has been advocated in the literature, it has been found to be of no benefit, painful, and potentially dangerous (24).

6. Do not give morphine, codeine, or meperidine (Demerol). These drugs seem to have a synergistic effect with the venom (20).

7. In case of arteriospasm, marked relief will be obtained with regional blocks using lidocaine (Xylocaine), (20). Lidocaine also seems to decrease the toxicity of the venom. Observe the extremity and continue the regional blocks as needed.

8. In extreme cases, an antivenin is available from The Poisonous Animal Research Laboratory, Tempe, Arizona (telephone 602-965-3536, Monday through Friday, 8:00 A.M.–4:30 P.M. At other times telephone the security department, 602-965-3456), (46).

SNAKE DESCRIPTIONS

Color is too variable to be of much use in identification of snakes. Patterns of markings are more reliable. The following are descriptions of a number of varieties of the genera *Crotalus* and *Bothrops*.

EASTERN DIAMONDBACK RATTLESNAKE (CROTALUS ADAMANTEUS).
Dark green or brown, with dark diamonds on the back and a cream to gray belly. The diamonds have a yellow edge and a light center.

WESTERN DIAMONDBACK RATTLESNAKE (CROTALUS ATROX).
Brown or gray, with black, white, and gray rings on the tail and two light stripes on the head. The diamonds on the back are indistinct and look like blurry ovals.

TIMBER RATTLESNAKE (CROTALUS HORRIDUS).
Gray or brown, with dark chevrons on the back. Some snakes are completely black.

RED DIAMONDBACK RATTLESNAKE (CROTALUS RUBER).
Similar to the western diamondback but has a reddish color.

MOJAVE RATTLESNAKE (CROTALUS SCUTULATUS).
Similar to the western diamondback except that the narrow dark rings on the tail are separated by wide light bands. *Identification is important because the venom is chiefly neurotoxic, and more antivenom is required. Bites may not appear serious until respiratory arrest occurs. The grading chart (Table 2) does not apply to bites of this snake.*

PACIFIC RATTLESNAKE (CROTALUS VIRIDIS OREGANUS).
Dark gray, olive, or brown, with diamonds or hexagonal

blotches on the back. Wide dark rings separated by narrow white ones on the tail.

GREAT BASIN RATTLESNAKE (CROTALUS VIRIDIS LUTOSUS).
Buff, light gray, or yellow. The back has dark crossblotches that may have light centers.

PRAIRIE RATTLESNAKE (CROTALUS VIRIDIS VIRIDIS).
Greenish gray to olive brown. The back has dark blotches with light edges.

SIDEWINDER RATTLESNAKE (CROTALUS CERASTES).
Light tan, gray, or pink, with dark spots and rings on the tail. An elevated scale above the eyes looks like a horn.

MEXICAN WEST COAST RATTLESNAKE (CROTALUS BASILICUS).
Brown or olive gray, with a dark tail and a white or yellow belly. The back has dark diamonds with light borders.

BARBA AMARILLA (BOTHROPS ATROX).
Olive green, gray, or brown, with a black stripe from the eye to the neck and a yellow chin and throat. The back is mottled or irregularly patterned, and the sides have a complex pattern of light-edged triangular blotches. Sometimes incorrectly called the fer-de-lance.

URUTU (BOTHROPS ALTERNATUS).
Brown, with a distinctive telephone-shaped mark edged in yellow on each side.

JARARACA (BOTHROPS JARARACA).
Olive green or brown, with a yellow-gray belly. Brown triangles edged in yellow on the sides, becoming rounded toward the tail.

JARARACA PINTADA (WAGLERS PIT VIPER)
(BOTHROPS NEUWIEDI WAGLA).
Reddish, olive, or brown, with a yellow belly. There is a double row of dark triangles connected in the center of the back, making a series of Xs. Dark spots sometimes alternate with the triangles.

JARARACUSSU (BOTHROPS JARARACUSSU).
Dull black head and body, with a yellow belly. Black triangles ringed with yellow on the back.

FER-DE-LANCE (BOTHROPS LANCEOLATUS).
Found only on the island of Martinique. Brown head and a brown, olive, or gray body with a dark stripe running down the neck from behind the eye. Hourglass-shaped blotches down the back. The name is sometimes incorrectly used for the barba amarilla.

ANTIVENIN SOURCES

Some manufacturers of antivenin have already been mentioned. The following are manufacturers of snake antivenin in South America and Mexico.

ARGENTINA—Institute Nacional de Microbiologia
          Veley Sarsfield 563, Buenos Aires

BRAZIL—Instituto Butantan,
       Caixa
       Postal 65, Sao Paulo
       Instituto Pinheiros Productos Therapeuticos,
       Caixa Postal 951, Sao Paulo

COLOMBIA—Instituto Nacional de Salud
          Calle 57, Numero 8–35, Bogota, D.E.

VENEZUELA—Laboratorio Behrens
          Calle Real de Chapellin,
           Apartado 62, Caracas D.F.

MEXICO—Instituto Nacional de Higiene,
       Cxda. M. Escobedo No. 20
       Mexico 13, D.F.
       Laboratories MYC, S.A.,—
       Av. Coyoacan
       1707 Mexico 12, D.F.

In the United States antivenin is manufactured by Wyeth Laboratories, Inc., Marietta, Pa. Some of the more exotic antivenins are kept at the Ross Allen Institute, Silver Springs, Florida. Most zoos have antivenin for the snakes they keep. They also have a cross reference of available antivenins with other zoos.

ANNUAL ANTIVENIN INVENTORY REPORT

Attached is the first annual compilation of antivenins as inventoried by institutions participating in the American Association of Zoological Parks and Aquariums Antivenin Index Center. This compilation provides (1) an inventory of antivenins, listed alphabetically by genus and species for which the antivenin is applicable and (2) participating institutions, personnel and day and night telephone numbers. The information is correct as of 1 July 1971 and will be updated regularly.

ANTIVENIN INDEX CENTER

The Antivenin Index Center is a current catalog of snake-bite antivenins stocked in North American zoos, laboratories and related institutions. The Center provides a 24 hour-a-day retrieval service on antivenins available for the treatment of venomous snake-bite from native and exotic species. The Index is limited to sera currently stocked by participating institutions. Also, full data is provided on telephone numbers and personnel to obtain emergency supplies of antivenins.

The Center *does not* stock antivenin; rather, it serves as an index for emergency *information* on available antivenins.

To Use This Service . . .

(1) Obtain both the *scientific name* (genus and species) and the *common or vernacular name* of the snake involved (e.g., *Dendroaspis polylepis*, Black mamba). Knowledge of the correct scientific name is almost indispensable in the proper selection of the appropriate antivenin.

(2) Call the Antivenin Index Center in Oklahoma City, 405-427-6232, for the following information:

- Antivenins applicable to your snake-bite which are currently stocked in North American institutions.

- Locations of available stocks nearest to you, amounts currently in stock and expiration dates.

- Emergency telephone numbers and names of key personnel for obtaining the antivenins from the listed institutions.

(3) Contact your nearest supply and make arrangements for emergency delivery of antivenin.

Used with the permission of the Oklahoma Poison Information Center, the Oklahoma City Zoo, and the American Association of Zoological Parks and Aquariums.

The following is a complete listing of antivenin inventories as carried by the Antivenin Index Center as of July 1, 1971. The listing is compiled alphabetically by the genus and species for which the manufacturer claims antivenin effectiveness.

Further, listed alphabetically by state, city and/or institution is the manufacturer's name, antivenin and amount (in cc's) as inventoried on July 1, 1971.

ACANTHOPUS ANTARCTICUS (Death adder)

California
    Los Angeles Lab   Cmw./Death adder/10
                                    Cmw./Poly./10
    Los Angeles Zoo   Cmw./Poly./20
    San Diego   Cmw./Death adder/50
    San Francisco   Cmw./Death adder/6,000 u
    Sacramento   Cmw./Death adder/12,000 u
Florida
    Silver Springs   Cmw./Death adder/36,000 u
Georgia
    Atlanta   Cmw./Death adder/60
                                      Cmw./Poly./60
Illinois
    Brookfield   Cmw./Death adder/12,000 u
Michigan
    Detroit   Cmw./Death adder/30,000 u
Texas
    Dallas   Cmw./Death adder/100
    Fort Worth   Cmw./Death adder/40
    Houston   Cmw./Death adder/40

AGKISTRODON ACUTUS (Sharp-nosed pit viper)

California
    Sacramento   Taiwan/Agkistrodon/120
    San Diego   Taiwan/Akgistrodon/80
    San Francisco   Taiwan/Agkistrodon/60
Georgia
    Atlanta   Taiwan/Agkistrodon/60
Ohio
    Cincinnati   Taiwan/Agkistrodon/60

AGKISTRODON HALSY (Halsy viper, mamushi)

California
    Los Angeles Zoo   IID Tokyo/Mamushi/60
Georgia
    Atlanta   Iran/Poly.Iran/120
                          IID Tokyo/Mamushi/60

District of Columbia
    Washington   IID Tokyo/Mamushi/50
Illinois
    Brookfield   Iran/Poly/80
New York
    Buffalo St. Univ.   Iran/Poly./100

AGKISTRODON RHODOSTOMA (Malayan pit viper)

California
    Los Angeles Lab   Pasteur/Ancistrodon/10
    Los Angeles Zoo   Thai/Pit viper/60
    Sacramento   Thai/Pit viper/60
Georgia
    Atlanta   Thai/Pit viper/60
Michigan
    Detroit   Thai/Pit viper/100
New York
    Bronx   Thai/Pit viper/100
Oklahoma
    Oklahoma City   Pasteur/Ancistrodon/60
Texas
    Dallas   Thai/Pit viper/70
    Houston   Thai/Pit viper/50
District of Columbia
    Washington   Thai/Pit viper/80

BITIS ARIETANS (Puff adder)
Use any antivenins listed for
BITIS GABONICA

BITIS GABONICA (Gaboon viper)

Alabama
    Birmingham   Behring/C. Africa/80
California
    Los Angeles Lab   CAPS/Poly./60
                          Pasteur/Bitis/20
                          Pasteur/Bitis–Echis/10
                          Pasteur/Bitis–Naja/20
                          Pasteur/Bitis–Echis–Naja/20
                          SAIMR/Trop./Poly./90
    Los Angeles Zoo   SAIMR/Trop./Poly./60
                          Behring/N. Africa & West/60
    Sacramento   SAIMR/Trop./Poly./60
    San Diego   Pasteur/Bitis/80
    San Francisco   SAIMR/Trop./Poly./60
    Saugus   SAIMR/Trop./Poly./30
District of Columbia
    Washington   Behring/C. Africa/140
                          Pasteur/Bitis–Echis–Naja/200
                          Pasteur/Bitis/100
                          SAIMR/Trop./Poly./40

Florida
    Silver Springs   SAIMR/Trop./Poly./110

Georgia
    Atlanta   Behring/C. Africa/150
                                    Pasteur/Bitis–Echis–Naja/60
                                    SAIMR/Trop./Poly./70
                                    Behring/N. Africa/180

Illinois
    Brookfield   Behring/C. Africa/80
                                    SAIMR/Trop./Poly./60
    Lincoln Park   Behring/C. Africa/60
                                    SAIMR/Trop.Poly./90

Kansas
    Topeka   Pasteur/Bitis/30
Louisiana
    Monroe   Behring/C. Africa/100
Maryland
    Baltimore   Pasteur/Bitis–Echis–Naja/170
                                      SAIMR/Trop./Poly./10
    Thurmont   SAIMR/Trop./Poly./20
Michigan
    Detroit   SAIMR/Trop./Poly./100
Missouri
    St. Louis   Behring/C. Africa/60
New York
    Bronx   CAPS/Trop./Poly./80
                                      SAIMR/Trop./Poly./70
    Buffalo Zoo   Behring/C. Africa/120
                                      Behring/N. Africa & West/120
                                    SAIMR/Trop./Poly./240
                                    Behring/C. Africa/60
    Rochester   SAIMR/Trop./Poly./60
                                      Behring/Europe/60
    Staten Island   SAIMR/Trop./Poly./100
Ohio
    Cincinnati   Fitz./Poly./160
    Columbus   Behring/C. Africa/60
                                      Behring/N. Africa/30
                                    Fitz./Poly./60
                                    SAIMR/Trop./Poly./60
Oklahoma
    Oklahoma City   Behring/Trop./Africa/110
                                    Pasteur/Bitis–Echis–Naja/50
    Tulsa   SAIMR/Trop./Poly./80
Pennsylvania
    Pittsburgh   Behring/Trop./Africa/60
                                    SAIMR/Trop./Poly./60
    Philadelphia   Pasteur/Bitis–Echis–Naja/150
                                    SAIMR/Naja–Bitis/200
                                    SAIMR/Naja–Bitis–Echis/100
South Dakota
    Rapid City   Behring/C. Africa/60
Texas
    Dallas   Behring/C. Africa/100
                                    Behring/N. Africa/50
                                    Pasteur/Bitis/100
                                    SAIMR/Trop./Poly./100
    Fort Worth   Behring/N. Africa/70
                                    SAIMR/Trop./Poly./120
    Victoria   SAIMR/Trop./Poly./40
    Waco   Behring/C. Africa/40

Washington
  Seattle   Fitz./Poly./40
Wisconsin
  Milwaukee   Behring/C. Africa/60
                       Pasteur/Bitis/150

BITIS NASICORNIS (Rhino viper)
Use any antivenin listed for
BITIS GABONICA

BOTHROPS ALTERNATA (Urutu)
California
  Hermosa Beach   Pinheiros/Antibothropico/50
  Los Angeles Lab   Butantan/Antibotropico/40
  Los Angeles Zoo   Butantan/Antibotropico/60
                       Behring/C. & S. America/60
  Sacramento   Butantan/Antiophidico/60
  San Diego   Butantan/Antibotropico/80
Georgia
  Atlanta   Behring/C. & S. America/60
                       Butantan/Antibotropico/70
Illinois
  Brookfield   Butantan/Antibotropico/80
Louisiana
  Monroe   Behring/C. & S. America/100
Michigan
  Detroit   Butantan/Antiophidico/150
Missouri
  St. Louis   Butantan/Antibotropico/60
New York
  Bronx   Butantan/Antibotropico/60
  Buffalo   Behring/C. & S. America/120
  Staten Island   Butantan/Antibotropico/60
Ohio
  Columbus   Behring/C. & S. America/30
Oklahoma
  Oklahoma City   Butantan/Antibotropico/60
Texas
  Dallas   Behring/C. & S. America/100
  Fort Worth   Behring/C. & S. America/50
  Houston   Pinheiros/Antibotropico/60
Utah
  Salt Lake City   Butantan/Antibotropico/30
                       Butantan/Antiophidico/40
  Also see North American Crotalids

BOTHROPS ATROX (Fer de Lance)
Florida
  Silver Springs   Costa Rica/Poly./20
Illinois
  Brookfield   Costa Rica/Poly./60
Indiana
  Indianapolis   Costa Rica/Poly./30
Also use any of the antivenins listed for
BOTHROPS ALTERNATA

BOTHROPS COTIARA (Cotiara)
Use any antivenins listed for
BOTHROPS ALTERNATA

BOTHROPS JARARACA (Jararaca)
Use any of the antivenins listed for
BOTHROPS ALTERNATA

BOTHROPS NEUWIEDI (Wied's lance-head)

California
 Los Angeles Zoo   Behring/C. & S. America/60
Georgia
 Atlanta   Behring/C. & S. America/60
Louisiana
 Monroe   Behring/C. & S. America/100
New York
 Buffalo Zoo   Behring/C. & S. America/120
Ohio
 Columbus   Behring/C. & S. America/30
Texas
 Dallas   Behring/C. & S. America/100

BUNGARUS CAERULEUS (Blue krait)

California
 Los Angeles Lab   Haffkine/Poly./30
 Los Angeles Zoo   Haffkine/Poly./60
 Sacramento   Haffkine/Poly./60
District of Columbia
 Washington   Haffkine/Poly./100
Georgia
 Atlanta   Kasauli/Poly./140
Illinois
 Brookfield   Haffkine/Poly./100
Kentucky
 Ft. Knox   Haffkine/Poly./340
Maryland
 Baltimore   Haffkine/Poly./60
 Thurmont   Haffkine/Poly./10
Missouri
 St. Louis   Kasauli/Poly./60
New York
 Bronx   Haffkine/Poly./60
 Buffalo   Haffkine/Poly./40
 Rochester   Haffkine/Poly./60
Texas
 Dallas   Haffkine/Poly./100
Washington
 Seattle   Haffkine/Poly./100

BUNGARUS FASCIATUS (Banded krait)

California
 Los Angeles Lab   Haffkine/Poly./30
 Los Angeles Zoo   Haffkine/Poly./60
         Thai/Banded krait/60
District of Columbia
 Washington   Haffkine/Poly./100
Florida
 Silver Springs   Thai/Banded krait/40
Georgia
 Atlanta   Thai/Banded krait/60
Illinois
 Brookfield   Haffkine/Poly./100
         Iran/Poly./80
         Thai/Banded krait/80

Kentucky
  Ft. Knox   Haffkine/Poly./340
Maryland
  Baltimore   Haffkine/Poly./60
  Thurmont   Haffkine/Poly./10
Michigan
  Detroit   Thai/Banded krait/100
New York
  Bronx   Haffkine/Poly./60
                              Thai/Banded krait/80
  St. Un. of Buff.   Iran/Poly./100
  Buffalo Zoo   Haffkine/Poly./40
  Rochester   Haffkine/Poly./60
Oklahoma
  Oklahoma City   Thai/Banded krait/100
Ohio
  Toledo   Thai/Banded krait/20
Pennsylvania
  Philadelphia   Thai/Banded krait/50
Texas
  Dallas   Haffkine/Poly./100
                              Thai/Banded krait/250
Washington
  Seattle   Haffkine/Poly./100
Wisconsin
  Milwaukee   Thai/Banded krait/100

BUNGARUS MULTICINCTUS (Formosan krait)

California
  Sacramento   Taiwan/Bungarus/120
  San Francisco   Taiwan/Bungarus/60
Georgia
  Atlanta   Taiwan/Bungarus, Naja/60
New York
  Rochester   Taiwan/Bungarus, Naja/60

CAUSUS RHOMBEATUS (Common night adder)

California
  Los Angeles Zoo   Behring/N. & W. Africa/60
Georgia
  Atlanta   Behring/N. & W. Africa/180
New York
  Buffalo Zoo   Behring/N. & W. Africa/120
Ohio
  Columbus   Behring/N. & W. Africa/30
Texas
  Dallas   Behring/N. & W. Africa/50
  Fort Worth   Behring/N. & W. Africa/70

CERASTES CERASTES (Horned viper)

Alabama
  Birmingham   Behring/N. & M. East/80
California
  Los Angeles Lab   Pasteur/Cerastes/20
  Los Angeles Zoo   Behring/N. Africa & West/60
Georgia
  Atlanta   Behring/N. Africa/60
                              Pasteur D'Algeria/Anti-viperin/60
Illinois
  Lincoln Park   Behring/N. & M. East/30

Michigan
    Detroit   Pasteur/Cerastes/100
New York
    Buffalo Zoo   Behring/N. Africa/120
Ohio
    Columbus   Behring/N. Africa/30
Oklahoma
    Oklahoma City   Behring/N. & M. East/60
Pennsylvania
    Philadelphia   Pasteur/Cerastes/10
Texas
    Dallas   Pasteur/Cerastes/50
    Fort Worth   Pasteur/Cerastes/70

CERASTES VIPERA (Avicanna viper)

Use any antivenin listed for
CERASTES CERASTES

CROTALUS ADAMANTEUS (Eastern diamondback rattlesnake)
    and others of the *Crotalus, Sistrurus* genera—

See North American Crotalids

CROTALUS DURISSUS (Tropical rattlesnake)

California
    Los Angeles Lab   Butantan/Anticrotalico/10
    Los Angeles Zoo   Butantan/Anticrotalico/180
                     Behring/C. & S. America/60
    Sacramento   Butantan/Antiophidico/60
    San Diego   Butantan/Anticrotalico/80
Florida
    Silver Springs   Costa Rica Poly./20
Georgia
    Atlanta   Behring/C. & S. America Poly./60
                     Butantan/Anticrotalico/70
Illinois
    Brookfield   Butantan/Anticrotalico/60
                     Costa/Rica/Poly./60
    Lincoln Park   Butantan/Anticrotalico/50
Indiana
    Indianapolis   Costa/Rica/Poly./30
Louisiana
    Monroe   Behring/C. & S. America/100
Michigan
    Detroit   Butantan/Anticrotalico/100
                     Butantan/Antiophidico/150
Missouri
    St. Louis   Butantan/Anticrotalico/60
New York
    Bronx   Butantan/Anticrotalico/60
    Buffalo   Behring/C. & S. America/120
    Staten Island   Butantan/Anticrotalico/60
Ohio
    Columbus   Behring/C. & S. America/30
Oklahoma
    Oklahoma City   Mex–INH/Anticrotalico/100
Texas
    Dallas   Behring/C. & S. America/100
    Fort Worth   Behring/C. & S. America/50
    Houston   Pinheiros/Bothrops–Crotalus/60

Utah
  Salt Lake City   Butantan/Antiophidico/40
Wisconsin
  Milwaukee   Butantan/Anticrotalico/50

DEMANSIA TEXTILIS (Brown snake)

California
  Los Angeles Lab   Cmw./Brown snake/10
                              Cmw./Poly./10
  Los Angeles Zoo   Cmw./Poly./20
  San Diego   Cmw./Brown snake/50
  San Francisco   Cmw./Brown snake/3.000 u
Georgia
  Atlanta   Cmw./Poly./60
Illinois
  Lincoln Park   Cmw./Brown snake/60
Michigan
  Detroit   Cmw./Brown snake/100
New York
  Bronx   Cmw./Brown snake/50

DENDROASPIS SP. (Mamba of questionable identity)
Use antivenins as listed for
DENDROASPIS VIRIDIS

DENDROASPIS AUGUSTICEPS (Green mamba)

Alabama
  Birmingham   Behring/C. Africa/80
California
  Los Angeles Lab   CAPS/Poly./60
                              SAIMR/Mamba/20
                              Pasteur/Dendroaspis/20
  Los Angeles Zoo   SAIMR/Mamba/60
  Sacramento   SAIMR/Mamba/60
  Steinhart   SAIMR/Mamba/60
District of Columbia
  Washington   Behring/C. Africa/140
Georgia
  Grant Park   Behring/C. Africa/150
                              SAIMR/Mamba/110
Illinois
  Lincoln Park   Behring/C. Africa/60
                              SAIMR/Mamba/100
  Brookfield   SAIMR/Mamba/90
                              Behring/C. Africa/80
Louisiana
  Monroe   Behring/C. Africa/100
Maryland
  Baltimore   SAIMR/Mamba/120
Michigan
  Detroit   SAIMR/Mamba/100
Missouri
  St. Louis   Behring/C. Africa/60
New York
  Bronx   Pasteur/Dendroaspis/100
                              SAIMR/Mamba/110
  Buffalo Zoo   Behring/C. Africa/120
                              SAIMR/Mamba/120
  Staten Island   SAIMR/Mamba/50
  Rochester   SAIMR/Mamba/60

Ohio
   Columbus Zoo   Behring/C. Africa/60
                             SAIMR/Mamba/50

Oklahoma
   Oklahoma City   Behring/C. Africa/110
Pennsylvania
   Philadelphia   Pasteur/Dendroaspis/10
S. Dakota
   Black Hills   Behring/C. Africa/60
Texas
   Dallas   Behring/C. Africa/100
                             SAIMR/Mamba/100
   Fort Worth   SAIMR/Mamba/70
   Waco   Behring/C. Africa/40
Washington
   Seattle   Fitz./Poly.–Mamba/40
Wisconsin
   Milwaukee   Behring/C. Africa/60
                             Pasteur/Dendroaspis/60
                             SAIMR/Mamba/140

DENDROASPIS JAMESONI (Jameson's mamba)

Alabama
   Birmingham   Behring/C. Africa/80
California
   Los Angeles Lab   Pasteur/Dendroaspis/20
                             SAIMR/Mamba/20
   Los Angeles Zoo   SAIMR/Mamba/60
   Sacramento   SAIMR/Mamba/60
   San Francisco   SAIMR/Mamba/60
District of Columbia
   Washington   Behring/C. Africa/140
Georgia
   Atlanta   Behring/C. Africa/150
                             SAIMR/Mamba/110
Illinois
   Brookfield   SAIMR/Mamba/90
                             Behring/C. Africa/80
   Lincoln Park   Behring/C. Africa/60
                             SAIMR/Mamba/100
Louisiana
   Monroe   Behring/C. Africa/100
Maryland
   Baltimore   SAIMR/Mamba/120
Michigan
   Detroit   SAIMR/Mamba/100
Missouri
   St. Louis   Behring/C. Africa/60
New York
   Bronx   Pasteur/Dendroaspis/100
                             SAIMR/Mamba/110
   Buffalo Zoo   Behring/C. Africa/120
                             SAIMR/Mamba/120
   Staten Island   SAIMR/Mamba/60
   Rochester   Behring/C. Africa/60
                             SAIMR/Mamba/60
Ohio
   Columbus Zoo   Behring/C. Africa/60
                             SAIMR/Mamba/50

Oklahoma
  Oklahoma City   Behring/C. Africa/110
Pennsylvania
  Philadelphia   Pasteur/Dendroaspis/10
South Dakota
  Black Hills   Behring/C. Africa/60
Texas
  Dallas   Behring/C. Africa/100
                           SAIMR/Mamba/100
  Fort Worth   SAIMR/Mamba/70
  Waco   Behring/C. Africa/40
Washington
  Seattle   Fitz./Poly–Mamba/40
Wisconsin
  Milwaukee   Behring/C. Africa/60
                           Pasteur/Dendroaspis/60
                           SAIMR/Mamba/140

DENDROASPIS POLYLEPIS (Black mamba)

Alabama
  Birmingham   Behring/C. Africa/80
California
  Los Angeles Lab   Pasteur/Dendroaspis/20
                           SAIMR/Mamba/20
                           CAPS/Poly./60
  Los Angeles Zoo   SAIMR/Mamba/60
  Sacramento   SAIMR/Mamba/60
  San Francisco   SAIMR/Mamba/60
District of Columbia
  Washington   Behring/C. Africa/140
Georgia
  Atlanta   Behring/C. Africa/150
                           SAIMR/Mamba/110
Illinois
  Lincoln Park   Behring/C. Africa/60
                           SAIMR/Mamba/100
  Brookfield   SAIMR/Mamba/90
                           Behring/C. Africa/80
Louisiana
  Monroe   Behring/C. Africa/100
Maryland
  Baltimore   SAIMR/Mamba/120
Michigan
  Detroit   SAIMR/Mamba/100
Missouri
  St. Louis   Behring/C. Africa/60
New York
  Bronx   Pasteur/Dendroaspis/100
                           SAIMR/Mamba/110
  Buffalo Zoo   Behring/C. Africa/120
                           SAIMR/Mamba/120
  Staten Island   SAIMR/Mamba/60
  Rochester   Behring/C. Africa/60
                           SAIMR/Mamba/60
Ohio
  Columbus Zoo   Behring/C. Africa/60
                           SAIMR/Mamba/50
Oklahoma
  Oklahoma City   Behring/C. Africa/110

South Dakota
  Black Hills   Behring/C. Africa/60
Texas
  Dallas   SAIMR/Mamba/100
  Fort Worth   SAIMR/Mamba/70
  Waco   Behring/C. Africa/40
Washington
  Seattle   Fitz./Poly. Mamba/40
Wisconsin
  Milwaukee   Behring/C. Africa/60
                              Pasteur/Dendroaspis/60
                              SAIMR/Mamba/140

DENDROASPIS VIRIDIS (Common mamba)

Alabama
  Birmingham   Behring/C. Africa/80
California
  Los Angeles Lab   Pasteur/Dendroaspis/20
Georgia
  Atlanta   Behring/C. Africa/150
Illinois
  Lincoln Park   Behring/C. Africa/40
  Brookfield   Behring/C. Africa/80
Louisiana
  Monroe   Behring/C. Africa/100
Missouri
  St. Louis   Behring/C. Africa/60
New York
  Bronx   Pasteur/Dendroaspis/100
  Buffalo Zoo   Behring/C. Africa/120
                              Behring/C. Africa/60
Ohio
  Columbus Zoo   Behring/C. Africa/60
Oklahoma
  Oklahoma City   Behring/C. Africa/110
South Dakota
  Black Hills   Behring/C. Africa/60
Texas
  Dallas   Behring/C. Africa/100
  Waco   Behring/C. Africa/40
Washington
  Seattle   Fitz./Poly. Mamba/40
Wisconsin
  Milwaukee   Behring/C. Africa/60
                              Pasteur/Dendroaspis/60

DISPHOLIDUS TYPUS (Boomslang)

California
  Los Angeles Lab   SAIMR/Boomslang/30
Illinois
  Brookfield   SAIMR/Boomslang/30
New York
  Bronx   SAIMR/Boomslang/30

ECHIS CARINATUS (Carpet viper)

Alabama
  Birmingham   Behring/N. & M. East/80

California
Los Angeles Lab   CAPS/Poly./60
                               Haffkine/Poly./30
                               Pasteur/Bitis–Echis/10
                               Pasteur/Echis–Naja/10
                               Pasteur/Echis/10
                               Pasteur/Bitis–Echis–Naja/20
                               SAIMR/Echis/20
Los Angeles Zoo   Behring/N. Africa & West/60
                               Iran/Echis/60
                               Haffkine/Poly./60
Sacramento   Haffkine/Poly./60
San Diego   Pasteur/Echis/60
San Francisco   Pasteur/Echis/60
District of Columbia
Washington   Pasteur/Bitis–Echis–Naja/200
                               Haffkine/Poly./100
Georgia
Atlanta   Behring/N. Africa/180
                               Kasauli/Poly./140
                               Pasteur/Bitis–Echis–Naja/60
Illinois
Brookfield   Behring/Viperin/60
                               Iran/Poly–India/80
                               Haffkine/Poly./100
Lincoln Park   Behring/N. & M. East/30
Kentucky
Fort Knox   Haffkine/Poly./340
Maryland
Baltimore   Haffkine/Poly./60
                               Pasteur/Bitis–Echis–Naja/110
Thurmont   Haffkine/Poly./10
                               Pasteur/Bitis–Echis–Naja/60
                               SAIMR/Bitis–Echis–Naja/20
Missouri
St. Louis   Kasauli/Poly./60
New York
Bronx   Haffkine/Poly./60
                               CAPS/Poly./80
                               Pasteur/Echis/60
Buffalo Zoo   Behring/N. Africa/120
                               Behring/N. & M. East/60
Rochester   Haffkine/Poly./60
St. Un. Buff.   Haffkine/Poly./40
                               Iran/Poly.–India/100
Staten Island   Pasteur/Echis/60
Ohio
Cincinnati   Haffkine/Poly./10
Columbus   Behring/N. Africa/30
Oklahoma
Oklahoma City   Behring/N. & M. East/60
                               Pasteur/Bitis–Echis–Naja/50
Tulsa   Behring/Viperin/100
Pennsylvania
Philadelphia   Pasteur/Echis–Bitis–Naja/150
                               SAIMR/Bitis–Echis–Naja/100
Texas
Dallas   Behring/N. Africa/50
                               Haffkine/Poly./100
                               Rogoff/Arabian Echis/50

Fort Worth   Behring/N. Africa/70
Waco   Behring/Viperin/40

ENHYDRINA SCHISTOSA (Common sea snake)

California
  Los Angeles Lab   Cmw./Sea snake/10
  Los Angeles Zoo   Cmw./Sea snake/30
  San Diego   Cmw./Sea snake/10
  San Francisco   Cmw./Sea snake/3,000 u
Georgia
  Atlanta   Cmw./Sea snake/60
Michigan
  Detroit   Cmw./Sea snake/60
Oklahoma
  Oklahoma City   Cmw./Sea snake/71.4
Pennsylvania
  Univ. Park   Cmw./Sea snake/60
Texas
  Dallas   Cmw./Sea snake/50

HEMACHATUS HAEMACHATUS (Ringhals cobra)

Alabama
  Birmingham   Behring/Cobra-Poly./80
                             Behring/C. Africa/80

California
  Los Angeles Lab   CAPS/Poly./60
                             SAIMR/Trop.Poly./90
  Los Angeles Zoo   SAIMR/Trop.Poly./60
  Sacramento   SAIMR/Trop.Poly./60
  San Francisco   Behring/Trop./60
  Saugus   SAIMR/Trop.Poly./30
District of Columbia
  Washington   Behring/C. Africa/140
                             SAIMR/Trop.Poly./40

Florida
  Silver Springs   SAIMR/Trop. Poly./110
Georgia
  Atlanta   Behring/C. Africa/150
                             SAIMR/Trop.Poly./120

Illinois
  Brookfield   SAIMR/Trop.Poly./60
                             Behring/C. Africa/80
  Lincoln Park   Behring/C. Africa/60
                             SAIMR/Trop. Poly./90

Louisiana
  Monroe   Behring/C. Africa/100
Maryland
  Baltimore   Behring/Cobra Poly./60
                             SAIMR/Trop. Poly./10

Michigan
  Detroit   SAIMR/Trop. Poly./100
Missouri
  St. Louis   Behring/C. Africa/60
                             Behring/Kobra/60

New York
  Bronx   Behring/Kobra/100
                             CAPS/Poly/80
                             SAIMR/Trop. Poly./70

Buffalo Zoo	Behring/C. Africa/120
	SAIMR/Trop. Poly./240
	Behring/C. Africa/60
Rochester	SAIMR/Trop. Poly./60
Staten Island	SAIMR/Trop. Poly./100
Ohio	
Cincinnati	Fitz./Poly./Trop./160
Columbus	Behring/C. Africa/60
	SAIMR/Trop. Poly./60
	Fitz./Poly. Trop./60
Oklahoma	
Tulsa	SAIMR/Trop. Poly./80
Oklahoma City	Behring/C. Africa/110
Pennsylvania	
Pittsburgh	Behring/Cobra Poly./60
	SAIMR/Trop. Poly./60
South Dakota	
Black Hills	Behring/C. Africa/60
Texas	
Dallas	Behring/C. Africa/100
	Behring/Cobra/50
	SAIMR/Trop. Poly./100
Fort Worth	Behring/Cobra Poly./110
	SAIMR/Trop. Poly./120
Victoria	SAIMR/Trop. Poly./40
Waco	Behring/C. Africa/40
Washington	
Seattle	Fitz./Poly. Trop./40
Wisconsin	
Milwaukee	Behring/C. Africa/60

HYDROPHIS CYANOCINTUS (Banded sea snake)

Use same antivenin as listed for
ENHYDRINA SCHISTOSA

LAEHESIS MUTA (Bushmaster)

California	
Los Angeles Lab	Butantan/Antilaquesico/10
Los Angeles Zoo	Butantan/Antilaquesico/60
San Diego	Butantan/Antilaquesico/80
San Francisco	Butantan/Bushmaster/60
Florida	
Silver Springs	Costa Rica/Poly./60
Georgia	
Atlanta	Butantan/Bushmaster/50
Illinois	
Brookfield	Costa/Rica/Poly./60
Lincoln Park	Butantan/Antilaquesico/50
Indiana	
Indianapolis	Costa/Rica/Poly./30
Missouri	
St. Louis	Butantan/Antilaquesico/60
Texas	
Dallas	Butantan/Antilaquesico/70
Houston	Pinheiros/Antibotropico/60
Utah	
Salt Lake City	Butantan/Antilaquesco/50

LAPEMIS HARDWICKII (Hardwick's sea snake)
New York
   Bronx   Pasteur–Viet Nam Lapemis/100

LATRODECTUS MACTANS (Black widow)
Georgia
   Atlanta   Merck/Lyovac/30
Illinois
   Lincoln Park   Merck/Lyovac/5.0
Kentucky
   Fort Knox   Merck/Lyovac/30
Louisiana
   Monroe   Merck/Lyovac/50
Ohio
   Cincinnati   Merck/Lyovac/10

MICRURUS CORALLINUS (Brazilian coral snake)
California
   Los Angeles Zoo   Butantan/Antielapidico/120
Florida
   Silver Springs   Butantan/Antielapidico/80
Georgia
   Atlanta   Butantan/Antielapidico/90
Illinois
   Brookfield   Butantan/Antielapidico/80
   Lincoln Park   Butantan/Antielapidico/50
Louisiana
   Monroe   Butantan/Antielapidico/110
Michigan
   Detroit   Butantan/Antielapidico/100
Missouri
   St. Louis   Butantan/Antielapidico/60
New York
   Bronx   Butantan/Antielapidico/200
Texas
   Dallas   Butantan/Antielapidico/100
   Fort Worth   Butantan/Antielapidico/120
   Houston   Butantan/Antielapidico/30
Utah
   Salt Lake City   Butantan/Antielapidico/30
Wisconsin
   Milwaukee   Butantan/Antielapidico/100
   Madison   Butantan/Antielapidico/100

MICRURUS FULVIUS FULVIUS (Eastern coral snake)
California
   Sacramento   Wyeth/Bivalent coral/50
   San Diego   Wyeth/Bivalent coral/50
District of Columbia
   Washington   Wyeth/Bivalent coral/10
Florida
   Silver Springs   Wyeth/Bivalent coral/50
Georgia
   Atlanta   Wyeth/Bivalent coral/50
Illinois
   Brookfield   Wyeth/Bivalent coral/50
Indiana
   Univ. Indianapolis   Costa Rica/Poly.coral/30
Louisiana
   Monroe   Wyeth/Bivalent coral/50

New York
  Bronx   Gennaro/Coral snake/40
Pennsylvania
  Wyeth Labs   Wyeth/Bivalent coral/
                                   supply adequate for demand

Ohio
  Cincinnati   Wyeth/Bivalent coral/10

NAJA HAJE (Egyptian cobra)

Alabama
  Birmingham   Behring/Cobra Poly./80
                                Behring/C. Africa/80
                                Behring/N. & M. East/80

California
  Los Angeles Lab   CAPS/Poly./60
                                Pasteur/Bitis–Echis–Naja/20
                                Pasteur/Naja/20
                                Pasteur/Echis–Naja/10
                                Pasteur/Naja/20

District of Columbia
  Washington   Pasteur/Bitis–Echis–Naja/200
                                Behring/C. Africa/140

Georgia
  Atlanta   Behring/C. Africa/150
                                Behring/N. Africa & West/180
                                Pasteur/Bitis–Echis–Naja/60

Illinois
  Brookfield   Behring/C. Africa/80
  Lincoln park   Behring/C. Africa/60
                                Behring/N. & M. East/30

Kansas
  Topeka   Pasteur/Naja/30
Louisiana
  Monroe   Central Africa/Behring/100
Maryland
  Baltimore   Behring/Cobra Poly./60
                                Pasteur/Bitis–Echis–Naja/110
                                Pasteur/Cobra/120
  Thurmont   Pasteur/Bitis–Echis–Naja/60
Missouri
  St. Louis   Behring/C. Africa/60
                                Pasteur/Cobra/120

New York
  Bronx   Pasteur/Naja/50
                                Behring/Cobra/100
  Buffalo   Behring/C. Africa/120
                                Behring/C. Africa/120
  Rochester   Behring/C. Africa/60
Ohio
  Columbus   Pasteur/Naja/60
                                Behring/C. Africa/60

Oklahoma
  Oklahoma City   Behring/N. Africa/30
                                Behring/C. Africa/110
                                Behring/N. & M. East/60
                                Pasteur/Bitis–Echis–Naja/60

Pennsylvania
  Philadelphia   SAIMR/Bitis–Echis–Naja/100
                                Pasteur/Naja–Bitis–Echis/150
  Pittsburg   Behring/Cobra Poly./60

South Dakota
   Black Hills   Behring/C. Africa/60
Texas
   Dallas   Behring/N. Africa/50
   Fort Worth   Behring/Cobra Poly./110
                       Behring/N. Africa/70
   Waco   Behring/C. Africa/40
Wisconsin
   Milwaukee   Behring/C. Africa/60

NAJA MELANOLEUCA (Forest cobra)

Alabama
   Birmingham   Behring/C. Africa/80
                       Behring/Cobra Poly./80
                       Behring/N. & M. East/80

California
   Los Angeles Lab   SAIMR/Trop. Poly./90
   Los Angeles Zoo   Behring/N. Africa & W./60
   Sacramento   SAIMR/Trop. Poly./60
   San Francisco   SAIMR/Trop. Poly./60
   Saugus   SAIMR/Trop. Poly./30
District of Columbia
   Washington   Behring/C. Africa/140
                       SAIMR/Trop. Poly./40

Florida
   Silver Springs   SAIMR/Trop. Poly./110
Georgia
   Atlanta   Behring/C. Africa/150
                       Pasteur/Bitis–Echis–Naja/60
                       SAIMR/Trop. Poly./70
                       Behring/N. Africa/180

Illinois
   Brookfield   Behring/C. Africa/80
                       SAIMR/Trop. Poly./60
   Lincoln Park   SAIMR/Trop. Poly./90
                       Behring/C. Africa/60
                       Behring/N. & M. East/30

Louisiana
   Monroe   Behring/C. Africa/100
Maryland
   Baltimore   Behring/Cobra Poly./60
                       Pasteur/Bitis–Echis–Naja/110
                       SAIMR/Trop. Poly./10
   Thurmont   Pasteur/Bitis–Echis–Naja/60
                       SAIMR/Trop. Poly./20

Michigan
   Detroit   SAIMR/Trop. Poly./100
Missouri
   St. Louis   Behring/C. Africa/60
                       Behring/Cobra/60

New York
   Bronx   Behring/Cobra/100
                       SAIMR/Trop. Poly./70
   Buffalo Zoo   Behring/C. Africa/120
                       Behring/N. Africa/120
                       SAIMR/Trop. Poly./240
                       Behring/C. Africa/60
                       Behring/N. & M. East/60
   Rochester   SAIMR/Trop. Poly./60
   Staten Island   SAIMR/Trop. Poly./100

Ohio
  Columbus   Behring/C. Africa/60
                                   Behring/N. Africa/30
                                   SAIMR/Trop. Poly./60

Oklahoma
  Oklahoma City   Behring/C. Africa/110
                                   Behring/N. & M. East/60
                                   Pasteur/Bitis–Echis–Naja/60
  Tulsa   SAIMR/Trop. Poly./80
Pennsylvania
  Pittsburgh   Behring/Trop. Africa/60
                                   Behring/Cobra/Poly./60
                                   SAIMR/Trop. Poly./60
  Philadelphia   SAIMR/Naja–Bitis–Echis/100
South Dakota
  Rapid City   Behring/C. Africa/60
Texas
  Dallas   Behring/C. Africa/100
                                   Behring/Cobra/50
                                   Behring/N. Africa/50
                                   SAIMR/Trop. Poly./100
  Fort Worth   Behring/Cobra Poly./110
                                   Behring/N. Africa/70
                                   SAIMR/Trop. Poly./120
  Victoria   SAIMR/Trop. Poly./40
  Waco   Behring/C. Africa/40
Wisconsin
  Milwaukee   Behring/C. Africa/60

NAJA NAJA (Asiatic cobra)

Alabama
  Birmingham   Behring/C. Africa/80
                                   Behring/Cobra/80

California
  Los Angeles Lab   CAPS/Poly./60
                                   Haffkine/Poly./30
                                   Pasteur/Cobra/30
  Los Angeles Zoo   Behring/N. & W. Africa/60
                                   Haffkine/Poly./60
                                   Thai/Cobra/60
  Sacramento   Haffkine/Poly./60
  San Francisco   Behring/C. Africa/60
                                   Thai/Cobra/60

District of Columbia
  Washington   Haffkine/Poly./100
Florida
  Silver Springs   Thai/Cobra/10
                                   Human antivenin for persons
                                     allergic to horse serum

Georgia
  Atlanta   Kasaula/Poly.–India/140
                                   Behring/C. Africa/150
                                   Pasteur/Cobra/60
                                   Thai/Cobra/60

Illinois
  Brookfield   Behring/C. Africa/80
                                   Iran/Poly.–India/80

Iowa
  Des Moines   Human antivenin

Kansas
  Topeka   Pasteur/Naja/30
Kentucky
  Fort Knox   Haffkine/Poly./340
                             Thai/Cobra/100

Louisiana
  Monroe   Behring/C. Africa/100
Maryland
  Baltimore   Behring/Cobra/60
                             Haffkine/Poly./60
                             Pasteur/Cobra/120
  Thurmont   Haffkine/Poly./10
Michigan
  Detroit   Thai/Cobra/200
Missouri
  St. Louis   Behring/Cobra/60
                             Behring/C. Africa/60
                             Kasauli/Poly./60

New York
  Bronx   Behring/Cobra/100
                             CAPS/Trop. Poly./80
                             Haffkine/Poly./60
  Buffalo Zoo   Behring/C. Africa/120
                             Behring/N. & W. Africa/120
  Buffalo St, Un.   Haffkine/Poly./40
                             Iran/Poly./100
                             Behring/C. Africa/60
                             Pasteur/Naja/60
  Rochester   Haffkine/Poly./60
                             Behring/C. Africa/60
                             Pasteur/Naja/60

Ohio
  Cincinnati   Haffkine/Poly./10
  Columbus   Behring/C. Africa/60
                             Behring/N. & W. Africa/30

Oklahoma
  Oklahoma City   Behring/C. Africa/110
                             Thai/Cobra/160
  Tulsa   Thai/Cobra/100
Pennsylvania
  Pittsburgh   Behring/C. Africa/60
                             Behring/Cobra/60
  Philadelphia   Pasteur/Cobra/110
Texas
  Dallas   Behring/C. Africa/100
                             Behring/Cobra/50
                             Haffkine/Poly./100
                             Thai/Cobra/50
  Fort Worth   Behring/Cobra/110
                             Behring/N. & W. Africa/70
  Waco   Behring/C. Africa/40
Utah
  Salt Lake City   Pasteur/Cobra/60
Washington
  Seattle   Haffkine/Poly./100
                             Pasteur/Cobra/50

Wisconsin
  Milwaukee   Thai/Cobra/90

NAJA NAJA ATRA (Taiwan cobra)

Georgia
   Atlanta   Taiwan/Naja–Bungarus/60
New York
   Rochester   Taiwan/Bungarus–Naja/60
Pennsylvania
   Philadelphia   Taiwan/Naja–Bungarus/60

Any antivenin listed for
NAJA NAJA should be of some value.

NAJA NAJAOXIANA (Oxus Riber cobra, Central Asian cobra)

California
   Los Angeles Zoo   Iran/Monovalent–Cobra/60
Georgia
   Atlanta   Iran/Poly.–Iran/60
Illinois
   Brookfield   Iran/Monovalent–Cobra/60
Pennsylvania
   Philadelphia   Iran/Monovalent–Cobra/100
Texas
   Dallas   Iran/Monovalent–Cobra/60

Any antivenin listed for
NAJA NAJA should be of some value.

NAJA NAJA PHILIPPINENSIS (Philippine cobra)

New York
   Rochester   Philippine/Cobra/100

Any antivenin listed for
NAJA NAJA should be of some value.

NAJA NIGRICOLLIS (Spitting cobra)

Alabama
   Birmingham   Behring/C. Africa/80
California
   Los Angeles Lab   CAPS/Poly./60
                          Pasteur/Bitis–Echis–Naja/20
                          Pasteur/Bitis–Naja/20
                          Pasteur/Echis–Naja/10
                          Pasteur/Naja/20
   Sacramento   SAIMR/Trop. Poly./60
   San Francisco   SAIMR/Trop. Poly./60
District of Columbia
   Washington   Behring/C. Africa/140
                          SAIMR/Trop. Poly./40
Florida
   Silver Springs   SAIMR/Trop. Poly./110
Georgia
   Atlanta   Behring/C. Africa/150
                          Behring/N. Africa/180
                          Pasteur/Bitis–Echis–Naja/60
                          SAIMR/Trop. Poly./70
Illinois
   Brookfield   Behring/C. Africa/80
                          SAIMR/Trop. Poly./60
   Lincoln Park   Behring/C. Africa/60
                          SAIMR/Trop. Poly./90
Louisiana
   Monroe   Behring/C. Africa/60

Maryland
  Baltimore   Pasteur/Bitis–Echis–Naja/110
                            SAIMR/Trop. Poly./10
  Thurmont   Pasteur/Bitis–Echis–Naja/60
                            SAIMR/Trop. Poly./20
Michigan
  Detroit   SAIMR/Trop. Poly./100
Missouri
  St. Louis   Behring/C. Africa/60
                            Behring/Cobra/60
New York
  Bronx   SAIMR/Trop. Poly/70
                            Behring/Cobra/100
  Buffalo Zoo   Behring/C. Africa/120
                            Behring/C. Africa/120
                            Behring/C. Africa/60
  Rochester   SAIMR/Trop. Poly./60
  Staten Island   SAIMR/Trop. Poly./100
Ohio
  Columbus   Behring/C. Africa/60
                            Behring/N. Africa/30
Oklahoma
  Oklahoma City   Behring/C. Africa/110
                            Pasteur/Bitis–Echis–Naja/60
                            Pasteur/N. & M. East/60
  Tulsa   SAIMR/Trop. Poly./80
Pennsylvania
  Philadelphia   Pasteur/Bitis–Echis–Naja/150
South Dakota
  Rapid City   Behring/C. Africa/60
Texas
  Dallas   Behring/C. Africa/100
                            Behring/N. Africa/50
                            SAIMR/Trop. Poly./100
  Fort Worth   Behring/N. Africa/70
  Waco   Behring/C. Africa/40
Wisconsin
  Milwaukee   Behring/C. Africa/60

NAJA NIVEA (Cape cobra)
Use any antivenin listed for
NAJA MELANOLEUCA EXCEPT for Behring/Near and Middle East.

NORTH AMERICAN CROTALIDS (Rattlesnakes, Moccasins)
Wyeth Crotalidae is believed to have all factors
important in the treatment of venoms from
BOTHROPS, SISTRURUS, AGKISTRODON CONTORTRIX and
AGKISTRODON PISCIVORUS as well as
CROTALUS.

Alabama
  Birmingham   Wyeth/Crotalidae/100
California
  Los Angeles Zoo   Wyeth/Crotalidae/60
  Fresno   Wyeth/Crotalidae/10
  Sacramento   Wyeth/Crotalidae/60
  San Francisco   Wyeth/Crotalidae/60
  Saugus   Wyeth/Crotalidae/30
District of Columbia
  Washington   Wyeth/Crotalidae/200

Florida
   Key Biscayne   Wyeth/Crotalidae/20
   Silver Springs   Wyeth/Crotalidae/140
Georgia
   Atlanta   Wyeth/Crotalidae/60
Illinois
   Brookfield   Wyeth/Crotalidae/50
   Lincoln Park   Wyeth/Crotalidae/80
Kansas
   Topeka   Wyeth/Crotalidae/10
Kentucky
   Fort Knox   Wyeth/Crotalidae/140
Louisiana
   Monroe   Wyeth/Crotalidae/80
Maryland
   Baltimore   Wyeth/Crotalidae/120
Michigan
   Detroit   Wyeth/Crotalidae/100
Minnesota
   St. Paul   Wyeth/Crotalidae/10
Missouri
   St. Louis   Wyeth/Crotalidae/60
New Jersey
   Mountainside   Wyeth/Crotalidae/50
New York
   Bronx   Wyeth/Crotalidae/70
   Buffalo Museum   Wyeth/Crotalidae/10
   Buffalo St. Un.   Wyeth/Crotalidae/50
   Buffalo Zoo   Wyeth/Crotalidae/160
   Rochester   Wyeth/Crotalidae/10
   Staten Island   Wyeth/Crotalidae/50
Ohio
   Cincinnati   Wyeth/Crotalidae/80
   Toledo   Wyeth/Crotalidae/30
Oklahoma
   Oklahoma City   Wyeth/Crotalidae/60
   Tulsa   Wyeth/Crotalidae/100
Oregon
   Portland   Wyeth/Crotalidae/90
Pennsylvania
   Philadelphia   Wyeth/Crotalidae/80
   Pittsburgh   Wyeth/Crotalidae/30
   Wyeth Labs   Supply adequate for demands
South Dakota
   Rapid City   Wyeth/Crotalidae/80
Texas
   Dallas   Wyeth/Crotalidae/120
   Fort Worth   Wyeth/Crotalidae/60
Utah
   Salt Lake City   Wyeth/Crotalidae/60
Washington
   Seattle   Wyeth/Crotalidae/10
Wisconsin
   Milwaukee   Wyeth/Crotalidae/100

NOTECHIS SCUTATUS (Tiger snake)

California
   Los Angeles Lab   Cmw./Poly./10
                            Cmw./Tiger snake/40

Los Angeles Zoo	Cmw./Poly./20
	Cmw./Tiger snake/60
Sacramento	Cmw./Tiger snake/12,000 u
San Diego	Cmw./Tiger snake/50
San Francisco	Cmw./Tiger snake/12,000 u
Florida	
Silver Springs	Cmw./Tiger snake/32,000 u
Georgia	
Atlanta	Cmw./Tiger snake/60
	Cmw./Poly./60
Illinois	
Brookfield	Cmw./Tiger snake/6,000 u
Lincoln	Cmw./Tiger snake/39.0
Michigan	
Detroit	Cmw./Tiger snake/30,000 u
Missouri	
St. Louis	Cmw./Tiger snake/60
New York	
Bronx	Cmw./Tiger snake/90
Rochester	Cmw./Tiger snake/18,000 u
Ohio	
Cincinnati	Cmw./Tiger snake/10
Pennsylvania	
Philadelphia	Cmw./Tiger snake/100
Texas	
Dallas	Cmw./Tiger snake/100
Fort Worth	Cmw./Tiger snake/40
Houston	Cmw./Tiger snake/70

"We would recommend Commmonwealth Tiger Snake for a King cobra bite."—Philadelphia Zoo

OPHIOPHAGUS HANNAH (King cobra)

Alabama	
Birmingham	Behring/Cobra Poly./80
California	
Los Angeles Lab	CAPS/Poly./60
	SAIMR/Trop. Poly./90
Los Angeles Zoo	SAIMR/Trop. Poly./60
	Thai/King cobra/60
Sacramento	SAIMR/Trop. Poly./60
	Thai/King cobra/60
San Diego	Thai/King cobra/80
San Francisco	Thai/King cobra/60
	SAIMR/Trop. Poly./60
Saugus	SAIMR/Trop. Poly./30
District of Columbia	
Washington	SAIMR/Trop. Poly./40
	Thai/King cobra/10
Florida	
Silver Springs	SAIMR/Trop. Poly./110
Georgia	
Atlanta	SAIMR/Trop. Poly./70
	Thai/King cobra/120
Illinois	
Brookfield	SAIMR/Trop. Poly./60
	Thai/King cobra/90
Lincoln Park	SAIMR/Trop. Poly./90
	Thai/King cobra/60

Maryland
  Baltimore   Behring/Cobra Poly./60
                           SAIMR/Trop. Poly./10
  Thurmont   Thai/King cobra/40
Michigan
  Detroit   SAIMR/King cobra/100
                           Thai/King cobra/200

Missouri
  St. Louis   Behring/Cobra/60
New York
  Bronx   Behring/Cobra/100
                           CAPS/Poly./80
                           SAIMR/Trop. Poly./70
                           Thai/King cobra/100
  Buffalo Zoo   SAIMR/Trop. Poly./240
                           Thai/King cobra/120
  Rochester   SAIMR/Trop. Poly./60
  Staten Island   SAIMR/Trop. Poly./100
                           Thai/King cobra/100

Ohio
  Columbus   SAIMR/Trop. Poly./60
                           Behring/N. & W. Africa/30

Oklahoma
  Oklahoma City   Thai/King cobra/100
  Tulsa   SAIMR/Trop. Poly./80
                           Thai/King cobra/160

Pennsylvania
  Philadelphia   Thai/King cobra/50
  Pittsburgh   Behring/Cobra Poly./60
                           SAIMR/Trop. Poly./60

Texas
  Dallas   Behring/Cobra/50
                           SAIMR/Trop. Poly./100
                           Thai/King cobra/100
  Fort Worth   Behring/Cobra Poly./110
                           SAIMR/Trop. Poly./120
                           Thai/King cobra/100
  Houston   Thai/King cobra/100
  Victoria   SAIMR/Trop. Poly./40
Wisconsin
  Milwaukee   Thai/King cobra/150

"We would recommend Commonwealth Tiger Snake
for a King Cobra bite."—Philadelphia Zoo

OXYURANUS SCUTTELLATUS (Taipan)

California
  Los Angeles Lab   Cmw./Poly./10
                           Cmw./Taipan/10
  Los Angeles Zoo   Cmw./Taipan/10
                           Cmw./Poly./20
  Steinhart   Cmw./Taipan/12,000 u
Georgia
  Atlanta   Cmw./Poly./60
Illinois
  Brookfield   Cmw./Taipan/6,000 u
Michigan
  Detroit   Cmw./Taipan/16,000 u
New York
  Bronx   Cmw./Taipan/20

PSEUDECHIS SPP. (Black snakes)

California
    Los Angeles Lab   Cmw./Papuan Black Snake/10
                                   Cmw./Poly./10
    Los Angeles Zoo   Cmw./Poly./20
Georgia
    Atlanta   Cmw./Poly./60
New York
    Bronx   Cmw./Black Snake/10

SYNANCEJA VERRUCOSA (Stonefish)

California
    San Francisco   Cmw./Stonefish/40

TRIMERESURUS FLAVOVIRIDIS (Habu)

California
    Los Angeles Zoo   IID–Tokyo/Habu/60
District of Columbia
    Washington   IID–Tokyo/Habu/10
Georgia
    Atlanta   IID–Tokyo/Habu/60
Texas
    Dallas   IMS–Tokyo/Habu/50
    Houston   IMS–Tokyo/Habu/40

VIPERA AMMODYTES (Sand viper)

Alabama
    Birmingham   Behring/Europe/80
District of Columbia
    Washington   Behring/Vipera/40
California
    Los Angeles Lab   CAPS/Poly./60
                                   Pasteur/Antiviperin E.O./20
                                   Pasteur/V. berusammodytes/10
                                   Pasteur/V. lebetineammodytes/20
    Los Angeles Zoo   Behring/Europe/60
    San Diego   Behring/Europe/80
Georgia
    Atlanta   Behring/Europe/150
                                   Pasteur/Antiviperin Trivalent/60
Illinois
    Brookfield   Behring/Viper/60
Kansas
    Topeka   Behring/Europe/30
Louisiana
    Monroe   Behring/Europe/100
Missouri
    St. Louis   Behring/Europe/60
New York
    Bronx   Behring/Europe/40
                                   CAPS/Trop. Poly./80
    Rochester   Behring/N. & M. East/60
    Staten Island   Behring/Europe/60
Ohio
    Columbus   Behring/Europe/30
Oklahoma
    Oklahoma City   Behring/N. & M. East/90
    Tulsa   Behring/N. & M. East/40

Texas
  Dallas   Behring/Europe/70
  Fort Worth   Behring/Europe/70
  Waco   Behring/Viper/40

VIPERA ASPIS (Jura viper)

Alabama
  Birmingham   Behring/Europe/80

Use same antivenin as applicable for
VIPERA AMMODYTES.

VIPERA BERUS (European viper)

Use same antivenins as applicable for
VIPERA AMMODYTES.

VIPERA LATASTI (Lataste's viper)

Use same antivenin as applicable for
VIPERA URSINII.

VIPERA LEBETINA (Levantine viper)

Alabama
  Birmingham   Behring/N. & M. East/80
California
  Los Angeles Lab   Pasteur/V. lebetina/20
                            Pasteur/V. lebetine-ammodytes/20
  Los Angeles Zoo   Behring/N. & W. Africa/60
                            Behring/Europe/60
                            Iran/Vipera lebetina/60
  San Diego   Behring/Europe/80
District of Columbia
  Washington   Behring/Europe/40
Georgia
  Atlanta   Behring/Europe/150
                            Behring/N. & W. Africa/180
                            Pasteur D'Algerie/Anti A.N. Viper/60
                            Iran/Poly./120

Illinois
  Brookfield   Behring/Europe/60
                            Iran/Poly./80
  Lincoln Park   Behring/N. & M. East/30
Kansas
  Topeka   Behring/Europe/30
Louisiana
  Monroe   Behring/Europe/100
Missouri
  St. Louis   Behring/Europe/60
New York
  Bronx   Behring/Europe/40
                            Pasteur/Viper–Near East/60
  Buffalo Zoo   Behring/N. & M. East/120
                            Behring/N. & W. Africa/120
  Buffalo St. Un.   Iran/Poly./100
  Rochester   Behring/N. & M. East/60
  Staten Island   Behring/Europe/60
Ohio
  Columbus   Behring/Europe/30
                            Behring/N. & East/30
                            Behring/N. & W. Africa/30

Oklahoma
  Oklahoma City   Behring/N. & M. East/60
  Tulsa   Behring/N. & W. Africa/100
Pennsylvania
  Philadelphia   Pasteur/Cerastes–V. lebetina/10
South Dakota
  Rapid City   Behring/Europe/40
Texas
  Dallas   Behring/Europe/70
                        Behring/N. & W. Africa/50
                        Iran/V. lebetina/60
  Fort Worth   Behring/Europe/70
                        Behring/N. & W. Africa/70
  Waco   Behring/Europe/40
Wisconsin
  Milwaukee   Behring/N. & M. East/100

VIPERA PERSICA (PERSIAN VIPER)

California
  Los Angeles Zoo   Iran/Persian viper/60
Illinois
  Brookfield   Iran/Persian viper/20
Georgia
  Atlanta   Iran/Poly. Iran/60

VIPERA RUSSELLI (RUSSELL'S VIPER)

California
  Los Angeles Lab   Haffkine/Poly./30
  Los Angeles Zoo   Haffkine/Poly./60
                        Thai/Russell's Viper/60
  Sacramento   Thai/Russell's Viper/60
                        Haffkine/Poly./60
  San Diego   Thai/Russell's Viper/60
  San Francisco   Thai/Russell's Viper/40
Florida
  Silver Springs   Thai/Russell's Viper/60
District of Columbia
  Washington   Haffkine/Poly./100
Georgia
  Atlanta   Thai/Russell's Viper/130
                        Kasauli/Poly./140
Illinois
  Brookfield   Iran/Poly–India/80
                        Haffkine/Poly./100
                        Thai/Russell's Viper/80
  Lincoln Park   Thai/Russell's Viper/30
Kentucky
  Fort Knox   Haffkine/Poly./340
Maryland
  Baltimore   Haffkine/Poly./60
  Thurmont   Haffkine/Poly./10
Michigan
  Detroit   Thai/Russell's Viper/100
Missouri
  St. Louis   Kasauli/Poly./60
New York
  Bronx   Haffkine/Poly./60
  Rochester   Haffkine/Poly./60
  Staten Island   Thai/Russell's Viper/60
  Buffalo St. Un.   Haffkine/Poly./40

Ohio
  Cincinnati   Thai/Russell's Viper/60
  Toledo   Thai/Russell's Viper/20
Oklahoma
  Oklahoma City   Thai/Russell's Viper/160
Pennsylvania
  Philadelphia   Thai/Russell's Viper/50
  Pittsburgh   Behring/Russell's Viper/40
Texas
  Dallas   Haffkine/Poly./100
                         Thai/Russell's Viper/50
  Fort Worth   Thai/Russell's Viper/50
Washington
  Seattle   Haffkine/Poly./100
Wisconsin
  Milwaukee   Thai/Russell's Viper/100

VIPERA URSINII

California
  Los Angeles Zoo   Behring/Europe/60
  San Diego   Behring/Europe/80
District of Columbia
  Washington   Behring/Europe/40
Georgia
  Atlanta   Behring/Europe/150
Illinois
  Brookfield   Behring/Europe/60
Kansas
  Topeka   Behring/Europe/30
Louisiana
  Monroe   Behring/Europe/100
Missouri
  St. Louis   Behring/Europe/60
New York
  Bronx   Behring/Europe/40
  Staten Island   Behring/Europe/60
Ohio
  Columbus   Behring/Europe/30
South Dakota
  Rapid City   Behring/Europe/40
Texas
  Dallas   Behring/Europe/70
  Fort Worth   Behring/Europe/70
  Waco   Behring/Europe/40

VIPERA XANTHINA PALESTINAE (Palestine viper)

Alabama
  Birmingham   Behring/Europe/80
California
  Los Angeles Lab   CAPS/Poly./60
  Los Angeles Zoo   Behring/Europe/60
  San Diego   Behring/Europe/80
Georgia
  Atlanta   Behring/Europe/150
Illinois
  Brookfield   Behring/Viper/60
Kansas
  Topeka   Behring/Europe/30
Louisiana
  Monroe   Behring/Europe/60

Missouri
  St. Louis   Behring/Europe/60
New York
  Bronx   CAPS/Trop. Poly./80
                            Pasteur/Viper–Near East/60
  Staten Island   Behring/Europe/60
Ohio
  Columbus   Behring/Europe/30
Oklahoma
  Tulsa   Behring/Viper/40
  Oklahoma City   Behring/Viper/60
Texas
  Dallas   Behring/Europe/70
                            Rogoff/Palestine viper/50
  Fort Worth   Behring/Europe/70
  Waco   Behring/Viper/40

WALTERINNESIA AEGYPTIA (Desert cobra)

Alabama
  Birmingham   Behring/Cobra/80
                            Behring/C. Africa/80
District of Columbia
  Washington   Behring/C. Africa/140
Georgia
  Atlanta   Behring/C. Africa/60
Illinois
  Brookfield   Behring/C. Africa/60
  Lincoln Park   Behring/C. Africa/60
Louisiana
  Monroe   Behring/C. Africa/100
Maryland
  Baltimore   Behring/Cobra/60
Missouri
  St. Louis   Behring/C. Africa/60
                            Behring/Cobra/60

New York
  Bronx   Behring/Cobra/100
  Buffalo Zoo   Behring/C. Africa/120
Ohio
  Columbus   Behring/C. Africa/60
Oklahoma
  Oklahoma City   Behring/C. Africa/110
Pennsylvania
  Pittsburgh   Behring/Cobra/60
South Dakota
  Rapid City   Behring/C. Africa/60
Texas
  Fort Worth   Behring/Cobra/110
  Waco   Behring/C. Africa/40
Wisconsin
  Milwaukee   Behring/C. Africa/60

LOCATION	INSTITUTION	NAME(s)	AREA CODE	TELEPHONES DAY	NIGHT
ALABAMA					
Birmingham	Jimmy Morgan Zoo	B. Truett	205	879-0408	879-0383
		J. Peavy			879-1818
CALIFORNIA					
Fresno	Roeding Park Zoo	P. Chaffee	209	266-8031	229-4965
		P. Alexander			227-3645
Hermosa	Hermosa Reptile and Wild Animal Farm	R. Folsom	213	376-5017	376-8697
		C. McClung		379-6322	379-5153
Los Angeles	Laboratory for Neurological Research	F. Russell	213	225-3115 ext. 7-2801	792-3670
Los Angeles	Los Angeles Zoo	N. Gale	213	666-4650	249-9881
		W. Turner			247-4819
Sacramento	Sacramento Zoo	R. Lacer	916	447-5094	457-4467
		K. Noblett			455-7466
		W. Meeker			447-2554
San Diego	San Diego Zoological Gardens	C. Shaw	714	234-5151	488-5953
		J. Staedeli			281-9644
San Francisco	Steinhart Aquarium	E. Herald	415	221-5102	755-5469
		K. Switak			586-1903 (213)-
Saugus	Africa, U.S.A., Inc.	M. Dinnes	805	259-1335	886-7273 (805)-
		R. Helfer			252-7188
DISTRICT OF COLUMBIA					
Washington, D.C.	National Zoological Park	J. Horsley	202	265-1868 ext. 234, 279 or 285	232-1752
		M. DePrato			(703)- 684-4947
		L. Schmeltz			(301)- 927-5163
FLORIDA					
Key Biscayne	Crandon Park Zoo	R. Sampsell	305	361-2515	361-5212
		G. Hubbell			361-5890

LOCATION	INSTITUTION	NAME(S)	AREA CODE	TELEPHONES DAY	NIGHT
Silver Springs	Ross Allen Reptile Institute	R. Allen	904	236-2858 236-2566	236-2866
		W. Gleason			236-2761
		A. Koukoulis			629-6176
GEORGIA Atlanta	Grant Park Zoo	J. Dobbs	404	627-5804 622-4839 628-2655	681-0194
		R. Hunt			627-3220 627-8695
ILLINOIS Brookfield	Chicago Zoological Park	R. Pawley	312	242-2630 485-0263	325-3256
		G. Rabb			442-9020
Chicago	Lincoln Park Zoological Gardens	L. Fisher	312	549-3000	327-4864
		S. Kitchener			878-3263
		E. Almandarz			761-4414
INDIANA Indianapolis	Indiana University Medical Center	S. Minton	317	264-7842	849-2596
IOWA Des Moines	Des Moines Children's Zoo	B. Elgin	515	283-4250	283-4034
KANSAS Topeka	Topeka Zoological Park	G. Clarke	913	272-5821	235-1651
		P. Linger			233-5786
		F. Kish			232-0891
KENTUCKY Fort Knox	US Army Medical Research Laboratory	R. Goellner	502	624-2952	351-6213 624-5246
LOUISIANA Monroe	Louisiana Purchase Gardens and Zoo	J. Yelberton	318	322-2479	323-2709
	St. Francis Hospital			325-2611	325-2611
MARYLAND Baltimore	Baltimore Zoo	A. Watson	301	889-9444	448-4366
		J. Groves			358-1465
Thurmont	Catoctin Mountain Zoological Park	R. Hahn	301	271-7488	271-7488
MICHIGAN Royal Oak	Detroit Zoological Park	R. Willson	313	398-0900	548-0318
		K. Kreag			588-3249
		J. Langhammer			541-3292
MINNESOTA St. Paul	St. Paul Como Park	J. Fletcher	612	488-3221	645-2496
		G. Pyhaluoto			488-1739
MISSOURI St. Louis	St. Louis Zoological Park	C. Hoessle	314	781-0900	353-5854
		D. Thompson			432-5568
NEW JERSEY Mountainside	Trailside Nature and Science Center	D. Mayer	201	323-5930	464-2568
		Union County Park Police		352-8431	352-8431

LOCATION	INSTITUTION	NAME(S)	AREA CODE	TELEPHONES DAY	NIGHT
NEW YORK					
Bronx	New York Zoological Park	W. King P. Brazaitia	212	933-1500	933-5586 (915)- 965-4740
Buffalo	Buffalo Museum of Science	R. Andrle	716	896-5200	649-5893
Buffalo	Buffalo Zoological Park	C. Freiheit M. Leumer	716	836-0711	833-0118 833-8738
Buffalo	State University of New York at Buffalo	C. Gans	716	831-2635 831-4838	835-3574
Rochester	Seneca Park Zoo	D. Michalowski F. Velte	716	266-6846	621-3467 266-2184
Staten Island	Staten Island Zoological Park	C. Kauffeld W. Summerville	212	442-3100	 356-7081
OHIO					
Cincinnati	Cincinnati Zoological Park	R. Lotshaw	513	281-0756 281-4700	683-1857
		E. Maruska B. Wakeman			931-4323 221-7837
Powell	Columbus Zoological Park	L. Pistoia J. Savoy	614	889-8335	885-6626 267-9470
Toledo	Toledo Zoological Society	D. Hipp C. Hardin	419	385-5721	693-8452 698-2251
OKLAHOMA					
Oklahoma City	Oklahoma City Zoo	L. Curtis H. Landreth D. Tuttle	405	424-3344	427-1901 424-3346 942-7983
Tulsa	Mohawk Park Zoo	D. Zucconi R. Sharpe J. Bennett	918	835-4221	627-0940 582-6749 936-5836
OREGON					
Portland	Portland Zoological Gardens		503	226-3646	
PENNSYLVANIA					
Philadelphia	Philadelphia Zoological Garden	K. Bowler	215	222-5300	(609)- 654-5868
Philadelphia	Wyeth Laboratories	M. Bierly E. Buckley	215	688-4400	666-0171 789-9798
Pittsburgh	Highland Park Zoo	W. Allen	714	661-1840 661-1844	242-1362
		H. Hays			242-6875
University Park	Department of Biology, Pennsylvania State Univ.	W. Dunson J. Hargleroad	814	865-2461	466-7259 865-6556
SOUTH DAKOTA					
Rapid City	Black Hills Reptile Gardens	E. Chace J. Campbell	605	342-5873	342-8569 342-1904
TEXAS					
Dallas	Marsalis Park Zoo	L. Calvin	214	946-5155 946-5154	224-1048
		J. Murphy G. Bullock J. Joy			948-6908 331-4916 371-3348

LOCATION	INSTITUTION	NAME(S)	AREA CODE	TELEPHONES DAY	NIGHT
Fort Worth	Fort Worth Zoological Park	E. Turner D. Brown J. Jones	817	923-4637	926-0476 924-0128 927-2104
Houston	Houston Zoological Gardens	J. Werler T. Logan	713	523-0149	665-1728 644-5839
Victoria	Victoria Zoological Park	G. Cook	512	573-4811 573-7681	575-6755
Waco	Central Texas Zoo	T. Granes	817	752-9101	753-6610
UTAH					
Salt Lake City	Hogle Zoological Garden	L. Farnsworth V. Barnes	801	322-1631	484-6624 484-1774
WASHINGTON					
Seattle	Woodland Park Zoological Gardens	F. Vincenzi C. Bradbury J. Nichols	206	782-5045	363-7089 783-6207 782-8456
WISCONSIN					
Milwaukee	Milwaukee County Zoo	G. Speidel R. Bullerman	414	771-3040	258-0444 425-2646
Madison	Reptiles Limited	L. Bernhardt	608	262-3886	

REFERENCES

1. Abbott, K. H. "Tick paralysis: A review." *Proceedings of the Staff Meeting of the Mayo Clinic* 18(1943):59.
2. Allen, F. M. "Observations on local measures in treatment of snake bite." *American Journal of Tropical Medicine* 19(1939):393–404.
3. Andrews, C. E., et al. "Venomous snake bite in Florida." *Journal of the Florida Medical Association* 55(1968):318–26.
4. Bierly, M. Z., and Buckley, E. E. "Treatment of crotalid envenomation." *Journal of the American Medical Association* 195(1955):575.
5. Block, M. J. "Function and operation of the facial pit of the pit vipers." *Nature* 165(1960):284–85.
6. Borden, J., et al. "Snakebite: Treatment by isolation perfusion technique." *Surgical Forum* 11(1960):186–87.
7. Costa, J. A. "Tick paralysis on the Atlantic seaboard." *American Journal of Diseases of Children* 83 (1952):336–47.
8. Dicus, D. R. "Treatment of poisonous snakebite." *Postgraduate Medicine* 31(1962):275–83.
9. Dillaha, C. J. "North American loxoscelism." *Journal of the American Medical Association* 188(1964):33–36.
10. Faust, E. C., and Russell, P. F. *Clinical Parasitology*, 7th Ed. Philadelphia: Lea & Febiger, 1964, pp. 986–87.
11. Gennaro, J. F. "Observation on treatment of snakebite in America." In *Venomous and Poisonous Animals and Noxious Plants of the Pacific Region*. New York: Macmillan, 1964, pp. 427–49.
12. Glass, T. G., Jr. "Snakebite." *Hospital Medicine* 7(1971):31–55.
13. Grant, M. C., and Henderson, L. J. "A summary of some previous accounts." *Iowa Academy of Science* 64(1957):686–97.
14. Handelman, N. I., and Zwemer, R. J. "Insect sting hypersensitivity and its management." *Journal of Kentucky Medical Association* 69 (1971):505–9.
15. Hershey, F. B., et al. "Surgical treatment of brown spider bites." *Annals of Surgery* 170(1969):300–8.
16. Horen, W. P. "Arachnidism in the United States." *Journal of the American Medical Association* 185(1963):839–43.
17. Insect Allergy Committee of the American Academy of Allergy. "Insect sting allergy." *Journal of the American Medical Association* 193(1965):109–14.
18. Revelations 9:1–10.
19. Klauber, L. M. *Rattlesnakes, Their Habits, Life Histories, and Influence on Mankind.* Berkeley: University of California Press, 1956.
20. Lowe, C. H., and Limbacher, H. P. "The treatment of poisonous bites and stings." *Arizona Medicine* 18(1961):128–31.
21. McCollough, N. C. "The juvenile amputee: Preliminary report of the problem in Florida." *Journal of the Florida Medical Association* 46 (1959):302–5.
22. McCollough, N. C., and Gennaro, J. F. "Evaluation of snake bites." *Journal of the Florida Medical Association* 64(1963):959–67.

23. McCollough, N. C., and Gennaro, J. F. "Summary of snake bite treatment." *Journal of the Florida Medical Association* 64(1963): 977.

24. McCollough, N. C., and Gennaro, J. F. "Coral snake bites." *Journal of the Florida Medical Association* 64(1963):968-72.

25. McCrone, J. D., et al. "Serological relationship of the lethal components of two black widow spider venoms." *Toxicon* 6(1968): 65-68.

26. Minton, S. A., Jr. "Venoms." *American Journal of Tropical Medicine* 6(1957):145-51; 1097-107.

27. Minton, S. A., Jr. "Venoms in desert animals." In *Desert Biology*, Vol. 1. New York: Academic Press, 1968, ch. 10, pp. 488-95.

28. Parrish, H. M. "Poisonous snakebites resulting in lack of venom poisoning." *Virginia Medical Monthly* 86(1959):396-401.

29. Parrish, H. M. "Death from bites and stings of venomous animals and insects in the United States." *Archives of Internal Medicine* 104 (1959):198-207.

30. Parrish, H. M., and Carr, C. A. "Copperhead bites in the United States." *Journal of the American Medical Association* 201(1967): 927-32.

31. *Poisonous Snakes of the World*. Washington, D.C.: Department of the Navy, Bureau of Medicine and Surgery, 1965, p. 68.

32. Rhoten, W. B. "Treatment of bite of a Mojave rattlesnake." *Journal of the Florida Medical Association* 55(1968):338-40.

33. Rose, I. "A review of tick paralysis." *Journal of the Canadian Medical Association* 70(1954):175-76.

34. Russell, F. E. "Snake venom poisoning." In *Cyclopedia of Medicine*, Vol. 2. Philadelphia: F. A. Davis and Company, 1962, pp. 199-210B.

35. Russell, F. E. "Poisoning." *American Journal of Medical Science* 243(1962):159-61.

36. Russell, F. E. "Letters to the editor." *Journal of the American Medical Association* 195(1966):596-97.

37. Russell, F. E. "Letters to the editor." *California Medicine* 106 (1967):248-49.

38. Russell, F. E. *Injuries by Venomous Animals*. National Clearinghouse for Poison Control Centers Bulletin, January-February, 1967.

39. Russell, F. E. "First aid for snake venom poisoning." *Toxicon* 4 (1967):285-89.

40. Smith, D. T., et. al. (Eds.) *Zinsser: Microbiology*, 12th Ed. New York: Appleton-Century-Crofts, 1966, p. 208.

41. Snyder, C. C., et al. "Study of snakebite." *Journal of the Florida Medical Association* 55(1968):330-37.

42. Sparger, C. F. "Problems in the management of rattlesnake bites." *Archives of Surgery* 98(1969):8.

43. Stahnke, H. L. "The effect of morphine and related substances on the toxicity of venoms." *American Journal of Tropical Medicine and Hygiene* 13(1964):346-51.

44. Stahnke, H. L. *The Treatment of Venomous Bites and Stings*. Tempe, Ariz.: Arizona State University, 1966, pp. 17-20; 32.

45. Stahnke, H. L. Personal communication.

46. Stahnke, H. L., et al. "Bite of the Gila monster." *Rocky Mountain Medical Journal* 67(1970):25-30.

47. Swaroop, S., and Grab, B. "Snakebite mortality in the world." *Bulletin of the World Health Organization* 10(1954): 35-76.

48. Taylor, E. H., et al. "Hemolysis, renal failure, and death, presumed secondary to bite of brown recluse spider." *Sourthern Medical Journal* 59(1966):1209-11.

49. Willson, P. "Snake poisoning in the United States." *Archives of Internal Medicine* 1(1908):516.

50. Wood, J. T. "Critique on "L-C" treatment of snakebites." *Southern Medical Journal* 49(1956):749-51.

51. Wood, J. T., Hoback, W. W., and Green, T. W. "Treatment of snake venom poisoning with ACTH and cortisone." *Virginia Medical Monthly* 82(1955):130-35.

52. Ya, P. M., and Perry, J. F., Jr. "Experimental evaluation of methods for early treatment of snakebite." *Surgery* 47(1960):975-81.

INDEX